RAW VEGANISM

HEALING DIET

Fully Explained

STAN SHEPHERD

Raw Veganism Healing Diet

Raw Veganism Healing Diet, Fully Explained. Copyright © 2018. All rights \reserved.

Cover design: Ljiljana Smilevski.

Contents

Dedication

To Jannette K. Shepherd, who introduced me to macrobiotics and started me on the road to raw vegan health.

Preface

As you read this book, you will take an exciting and inspirational journey into new realms of self-knowledge and self-awareness that will enable you to become a more energetic and effective person.

You will explore the basic laws of Nature and learn how to apply them for optimum health. You will understand how a detailed knowledge of foods and nutrition can enable you to become your own doctor using the untainted and unaltered foods of Nature.

Many of the things discussed in this book will perhaps be new and unfamiliar to you. But I assure you, everything has been proven and tested through personal experience.

The book will show you exactly how to rebuild yourself from the inside out, using the best building blocks that Nature can provide. It explains how diseases are healed through the amazing powers of living (raw) plant foods, and how health can be saved from being wrecked on other diets. It describes why the vegetarian and vegan diets cannot deliver true vibrant health.

This book is for anyone who is interested in improving their health. It is for the seeker of truth about foods and nutrition. It is for those who have many years ahead of them who want to remain healthy and enjoy the best out of life. It is for those who perhaps have no other choice than to begin learning about foods and nutrition at a late age, who realize that if they do not do something about their health then only worse days are ahead for them.

This book shares what I have learned about foods and nutrition over the years, and describes the amazing powers of raw plant foods to heal diseases, prevent diseases from taking root, and promote and maintain optimum health. The amazing powers of raw plant foods are made available to anyone who adopts the raw vegan diet.

If you are currently suffering from a health issue, or if your health is not up to par, then this book is for you. You don't have to be familiar with the vegetarian, or vegan, or raw vegan diets. This book will introduce them to you.

If you are already a vegetarian or a vegan, this book is also for you. It will greatly assist you in getting off those diets and going all the way to the raw vegan diet, the only diet that can give you the results that you are looking for.

The raw vegan diet is a complete shift in eating habits, away from lifeless cooked foods to living natural foods, the only foods that have the authentic life force properties that Nature intended for us to receive, and that support all bodily functions and contain the enzymes and nutrients the body needs to heal itself.

Introduction

"The rest of the world lives to eat, but I eat to live." - Socrates (470-399 B.C.).

Since the beginning of the 21st century, more people have switched to vegetarian and vegan diets for health reasons, such as degenerative diseases or the increasingly high levels of mercury in fish, than ever before. While vegetarian and vegan diets are healthier than the typical American diet, they do not go far enough in preventing the top 10 leading causes of death, or the degenerative diseases that are so prevalent in the world today.

Both the vegetarian and vegan diets restrict or avoid animal-based foods, which is to their benefit. However, both allow cooked foods to be eaten, which is to their detriment, as we shall see in this book, since cooked foods are harmful to human health.

The raw vegan diet is based on many studies by modern nutritional experts showing that substituting raw plant foods for cooked foods heals disease, prevents disease from taking root and promotes genuine health. Raw veganism incorporates this paradigm shift in nutritional thinking by excluding all cooked foods from the diet.

Practically speaking, what's more important than health? If you do not have health then you cannot accomplish the things you want to accomplish or need to do. What good is a million dollars if you are tied to a dialysis machine, or otherwise hindered from enjoying an active, healthy lifestyle because of a health issue?

Most people are concerned about their health. But very few will ever make the changes required to really improve their health. Eating prepared vegetables at the whole food stores, or reducing saturated fats and having a salad with a chicken sandwich will not cut it. You cannot achieve genuine health by making half-hearted attempts at trying to be healthy. That includes any partially-raw diet, like the vegan 80/20 diet (80% raw, 20% cooked) which I was on for a long time. It's like being partially well, which means partially unwell.

Actually, the vegan 80/20 diet amounts to being less than 80% well since cooked foods, which are permitted on the vegan diet, cause toxin buildup in the body tissues which further complicates health. There is no substitute for being 100% healthy. Eating 100% raw plant foods makes you 100% well. Anything short of that does not. These truths will be brought out and explained in this book.

Health issues uncommon in the past are frequently experienced today. Widespread and serious illnesses and diseases strike everyone, everywhere. How many people do you know who are suffering from a health affliction or disorder? How many of you reading this book have a health issue that you are wrestling with?

It has been my experience and observation that we are more than capable of causing our own sicknesses. We unwittingly bring sickness and disease upon ourselves through dietary practices that are contrary to the laws of nature. The body requires a variety of nutrients to keep itself in health, but seldom finds them in the foods that are commonly eaten. It requires enzymes for proper digestion, but they are destroyed by heat, and almost all refined and processed foods are heat treated. Deprived of the nutrients and other essentials it needs to enhance the body's self-cleansing process, the natural law of cause and effect determines the outcome, which is ill health.

The evidence against the foods that are most commonly eaten in this country is so overwhelming that it is surprising that anyone would continue to eat them, especially when there are so many other foods available that promote health, reduce the chances of getting diseases and provide the energy and stamina needed for an active, productive life.

I am convinced that the key to improving health is self-education about foods and nutrition. Without sufficient knowledge about foods and nutrition we remain wholly ignorant of how to achieve optimum health. The knowledge needed about foods and nutrition is best obtained by reading books, and utilizing other learning tools such as the Web, to discover the truth about these vital subjects.

"Get Wisdom! Get understanding!" - Prov. 4:5.

Before I began searching for answers about foods and nutrition, I ate the typical American diet. That was years ago. In the 1980s, based on the books that I read, I became aware of the health hazards of eating animal-based and man-made foods. I cut back on meat and most dairy products, weaned myself of sugary foods and drinks and became macrobiotic, eating mostly raw or cooked vegetables, including sea vegetables, and brown rice.

Then for over 20 years I was a vegetarian, eating mostly plant foods, but also some fish. When I gave up fish, I became a vegan (no animal-based foods), but I still ate cooked plant foods.

While on the vegan diet, my health stalled. It just stopped improving. And when health stops improving it typically starts to decline. I didn't know why my health wasn't improving, but I continued to search for the answers.

I continued to read about foods and nutrition. The books I read talked a lot about the importance of eating raw (uncooked) plant foods. Slowly, this new information began to sink in. When I became convinced of the dangers of eating cooked foods, I quit cooked foods and became a raw vegan. That was the best decision I ever made.

This book describes the raw vegan diet in detail. It is not a raw food recipe book. It is not about how to lose weight, or how to improve health through exercise, yoga or stress reduction. This book is all about the raw vegan diet, how to attain it and how to keep it. It explains what foods should be eaten, and why. It discusses the dangers of cooked and starchy foods. It provides the basics of proper food combining. It explains how living plant foods rejuvenate the body and heal disease. In this book, you will discover what raw veganism is, how to transition to the raw vegan diet from whatever diet you may now be on, and what to expect when you attain the raw vegan diet. Everything you need to know about getting to the raw vegan diet and staying on it is covered in this book.

For most people, the journey to optimum health will be a new experience, a journey into uncharted territory. I guarantee you it will be like no other. It is my hope that your journey will be as rewarding and satisfying as mine has been, and continues to be.

Raw Veganism

"Nothing is as powerful as an idea whose time has come." - Victor Hugo.

What is raw veganism? It is a diet, the raw vegan diet, which includes all raw (that is, uncooked) fruits and vegetables, leafy greens, nuts and seeds, grains and legumes, and Superfoods. These foods may be eaten in any quantity desired. It excludes all animal-based foods (animal products) and all cooked foods.

For comparison purposes, the plant-based diets are as follows:

Vegetarian Diet – The vegetarian diet is a diet that consists mostly of plant foods. It minimizes meat and dairy products but can include some fish, and/or some dairy and poultry such as cheese and eggs. The emphasis of the vegetarian diet is on eating mainly plant foods but also cutting back on animal-based foods. Both cooked plant and animal-based foods are allowed on the vegetarian diet.

Vegan Diet – The vegan diet is somewhat like the vegetarian diet but it goes further to exclude *all* animal-based foods, even fish, cheese and eggs. The vegan diet allows cooked plant foods to be eaten.

Raw Vegan Diet – The raw vegan diet is somewhat like the vegan diet in that it excludes all animal-based foods. But it also excludes all cooked foods, which includes cooked plant foods.

Cooked foods contain coagulated and unusable proteins and dead enzymes that are toxic to the body.

As stated previously, raw plant foods are foods as found in Nature. They are not cooked or chemically altered, and do not contain preservatives, artificial colors or flavors. Raw plant foods are living foods. Their natural life force properties are intact. It is this life force that is imparted to us when we eat raw plant foods.

What Foods Should We Eat and Why?

"He who does not know food, how can he understand the diseases of man?" - Hippocrates.

Much of what has been discussed in previous chapters provided reasons for avoiding certain types of foods and eating the right foods. This chapter explains more specifically what foods we should eat and why.

Increasing scientific evidence compiled every year links the top 10 leading causes of death, and the degenerative diseases so prevalent in the world today, to eating meat-based and dairy-based diets. These studies continue to show that people eating a plant-based diet have increased longevity and health compared to those eating a meat-based and/or dairy-based diet. Many books published in recent years provide the results of these clinical studies.

The China Study, published in 2005, may be the most comprehensive study of human nutrition ever performed. The population, or group, that was used in the study was the entire population of China. Written by T. Colin Campbell, a professor of Nutritional Biochemistry at Cornell University, and his son Thomas M. Campbell II, a physician, the study proved that whole plant-based foods, not animal-based foods, are the most beneficial foods for people. The study showed that people eating a plant-based diet have increased longevity and health compared to those eating a meat-based and/or dairy-based diet.

How Not to Die, written by Dr. Michael Greger and published in 2015, confirmed the conclusions of *The China Study*, and provided additional research and study results that emphasized the importance of eating plenty of whole plant foods, such as fruits and vegetables, to prevent and even *reverse* the chronic diseases of the Western world, including cancer, diabetes, heart disease and brain diseases.

The hazards of eating animal-based foods, or animal products, are well known to most educated people. Eating animal products causes plaque formations in the arteries, which is known to cause hardening of the arteries, which can lead to heart disease and stroke. Harmful mutagens and carcinogens, such as acrylamide, HCAs, PAHs and AGEs, are formed when animal products are cooked (for more detail, see Victoria Boutenko's book, *12 Steps to Raw Foods*). Animal products can contain nitrates, chlorine and ammonia and are susceptible to hosting various forms of life-destroying bacteria.

Studies conducted on animals and people show that blood cholesterol levels increase when animal protein is eaten. Dr. Caldwell Esselstyn, Jr., in his book, *Prevent and Reverse Heart Disease,* says that anyone with high blood cholesterol levels is prone to heart disease. Animal-based foods contain cholesterol, whereas no plant foods contain cholesterol. Dr. Esselstyn changed his diet to a plant-based diet and strongly recommended his patients to do the same. Those who did were able to cleanse their coronary arteries of plaque formations, which means their arteries were no longer clogged, and Dr. Esselstyn proved this by way of coronary angiograms.

Dr. Esselstyn is now a leading advocate of raw plant foods. He is featured in the food documentary DVD, *Forks Over Knives*. Testimonies given in that DVD attest to the powers of raw plant foods to heal a number of leading chronic diseases, including heart disease and breast cancer.

In *Fruits and Farinacea – The Proper Food of Man*, John Smith tells us that based on all accessible sources, our progenitors were frugivorous, i.e., fruit eaters. Both anthropological studies and studies of how the human body functions support this conclusion.

"Meat is not man's natural food, since he is not either a carnivorous or an omnivorous animal. Every argument drawn from comparative anatomy, from physiology, from chemistry, from experience, from observation, and, when rightly used, from common sense, all agree that man is not a meat-eating animal.

He can never be as healthy under the prevailing "mixed" diet as he would if he were to follow the dictates of Nature and live on his natural food – fruits and nuts, eaten in their uncooked, primitive form. Every element the system needs can be shown to be present in these foods, in their proper proportion, while, being live foods instead of mere "dead ashes", which is all the cooking process leaves, they will be found to supply a degree of vital life and energy which no cooked foods ever supplied or could supply."
- Hereward Carrington, Vitality, Fasting and Nutrition.

Human beings, in many key physiological ways, are not like other animals. We have hands with opposable thumbs, non-claw-like nails, teeth that are not suitable for tearing hide or flesh, or breaking bones, but rather for grinding plant foods, and long, not short, digestive tracts including 20-30 foot long intestines that are ideally suited for digesting fiber-rich foods like fruits, vegetables, nuts, seeds and grains.

David Wolfe in his book, *The Sunfood Diet Success System*, includes as Appendix A, an "Anatomy Chart" that identifies 17 physiological ways in which human beings are ideally suited for eating a plant-based diet. Websites also support this conclusion, as can be seen by searching on "Are humans frugivores?"

These studies show that humans are naturally suited for picking, chewing and digesting plant foods. Chimpanzees, which are very similar to humans physiologically, subsist almost entirely on fruits and greens.

According to the Bible, the first people on earth lived to very great ages. Adam lived to 930 years   Methuselah lived 969 years. Prior to the Flood, the average human lifespan was about 900 years. However, immediately after the Flood, when animal food was permitted to be eaten, the average lifespan fell to about 400 years. Later, when Jacob, the father of the twelve tribes of Israel, lived, the average lifespan was only about 150 years.

Based on the latest worldwide statistics from WHO, the average human lifespan is currently 72 years.

The worldwide increase in food production has resulted in a worldwide topsoil mineral deficiency. The topsoil in which plants are grown is now depleted of its minerals. Reports on the Web cover recent losses of nutrients in crops. Only decades ago, the same crops were richer in vitamins and minerals. Meat and dairy products (animal products) are affected even worse. Animals consume the mineral deficient crops and become mineral deficient. Cooking animal products further depletes them of minerals and vitamins.

The mineral deficiency of the topsoil is being blamed on improper farm management practices resulting in ill replenishment of the minerals back into the soil. The meteoric rise in food productivity and efficiency since the last century have not been balanced by a corresponding increase in the addition of nutrients back into the soil.

Nutritional deficiency occurs when the body does not absorb or get enough of the necessary amounts of nutrients it needs from foods. Nutrients include vitamins, minerals, proteins, carbohydrates, fats and water. They are essential for cellular growth and the maintenance of life. The body does not manufacture nutrients, but obtains them from the surrounding environment. We get most of our nutrients from foods.

People who eat the traditional American diet are nutrient deficient. This deficiency has been shown to be the cause of a number of serious health problems. To make up for the mineral-starved and vitamin-starved foods now being produced, many people take multivitamin/mineral supplements on the advice of their doctors. Billions of dollars are spent each year in America alone on these supplements.

Unfortunately, most of the multivitamin/mineral supplements are *inorganic* substances that cannot be utilized by the body. Studies have shown that these supplements provide little, if any, benefit to human health. See Web articles, such as from searching on "multivitamin/mineral supplements." It is also discussed in books by Dr. Ann Wigmore (see Bibliography), among others.

"Inorganic minerals are rejected by the cells of the body, which, if not evacuated, can cause arterial obstructions and even more serious damage." - Norman W. Walker, <u>Water Can Undermine Your Health.</u>

According to many nutritionists who are referenced in this book, the cells of the body can only utilize minerals that are in organic form, which is one of the reasons why plant foods are so important to us. Plants convert inorganic minerals found in the soil and water into organic form that is readily assimilated by the cells of the body.

Doctors often prescribe medication that is calcium carbonate based, which is an inorganic mineral compound. Calcium carbonate is the main ingredient in almost all antacids, and it is also found in some brands of aspirin.

The days when milk cows roamed the pastures and got their calcium from grass are over. Today's milk cows do not go outside to graze. They seldom move out of their stalls or feedlots. Their urine and feces are removed mechanically. Their milk is removed by machines hooked up to their udders. They get their calcium and other nutrients from their feed, which, according to Web articles, is a specially formulated mix of grains, soy, silage and inorganic calcium in the form of calcite flour (calcium carbonate), aragonite (calcium carbonate), crushed bones, and other bits and pieces of slaughtered animals to maximize weight gain and therefore profits when the cows are no longer useful as money-making machines. Apparently, calcium from cow's milk is mainly inorganic calcium.

On the raw vegan diet, there is no need for multivitamin/mineral supplements, since all the minerals and vitamins needed to support life are in raw plant foods in their proper organic form and undestroyed by heat. An example is the amount of organic calcium that is in collard greens. According to the USDA publication *Nutritive Value of American Foods*, just two-thirds cup of collard greens has 91% of the calcium in a cup of milk. Other plant foods having about the same amount of calcium are kelp and almonds.

A whole plant food diet also compensates for topsoil mineral deficiency since more plant foods are eaten on the diet. In addition, the diet includes sea vegetables, which are grown in the ocean – a mineral-rich environment.

Nutritional deficiency is so widespread in this country and in the world today that it can be said to be the number one health problem in the world, even among people who supposedly eat a healthy, balanced diet.

Excitotoxins are substances added to processed foods and beverages for the purpose of stimulating brain neurons. For years, the food industry has designed food products to titillate the taste buds and activate the reward centers of the brain. The diverse chemicals that are used for these purposes include excitotoxins. The term was popularized by Dr. Russel Blaylock in his book, *Excitotoxins, The Taste that Kills*. As stated in the book, these substances are found in almost all processed foods. Excitotoxins include monosodium glutamate (MSG)[1], aspartame (used in artificial sweeteners), cysteine (used in breads), hydrolyzed protein, and aspartic acid. These substances can stimulate brain neurons so severely that they are killed, resulting in varying degrees of brain damage.

Remember that piercing headache you got the last time you ate Chinese food? It was probably due to the MSG used on the food. The Web adequately covers the dangers of MSG, e.g., do a search on "msg in foods."

As of this writing, there are no regulations requiring the food industry to test its products for whether they cause brain damage or food addictions.

The deliberate tampering of foods to increase taste appeal at the expense of harming the body, while attesting to the inventiveness and ingenuity of the American spirit, typifies how low we have sunk in manipulating foods for financial gain.

---

[1] According to Blaylock's book, the food industry is on a quest to disguise MSG in foods. A list of common additives that contain MSG is found in the book.

It is entirely possible that the causative factor, or at least a major contributing factor, to the sharp rise in brain diseases in our culture, including dementia and other neurological disorders, is the continued use year after year of food products that contain excitotoxins. I recommend Dr. Blaylock's book to anyone. It includes a list of chemicals that should be tacked to our kitchen walls. It will make you check the foods labels all over again.

To avoid the hazards that have been described, and more (I'm sure I haven't mentioned all of them) we should eat raw plant foods. This is what nutritional experts have been telling us for years, as documented in their books listed in the Bibliography.

We live in the age of information, and the Web/Internet is our most popular information source. While I consider the Web a very useful tool for learning about foods and nutrition, it should not be our only source for this information. Much of what is on websites is opinion-oriented or provided in support of commercial interests. Opinions can run the gamut, and misrepresentation and conflicting information can be, and often times are, the result.

"As corrupting an influence as money is in medicine, it appears to be even worse in the field of nutrition, where it seems everyone has his or her own brand of snake oil supplement or wonder gadget. Dogmas are entrenched and data too often cherry picked to support preconceived notions." - Dr. Michael Greger, How Not To Die.

For example, for years leading nutritionists have contended that cooked and starchy foods are detrimental to human health, and that abstinence from such foods is necessary to cure health disorders including diseases. However, at the time of this writing, many of the websites queried for this information actually encourage eating cooked and starchy foods as part of a healthy diet.

We cannot trust everything we read on the Web. But that being said, the Web should not be ignored as a learning tool in self-education about foods and nutrition. However, for those of us who are seeking answers to the really tough questions of today about foods and nutrition, books provide the answers. The books that are listed in the Bibliography are excellent resources that will aid anyone in their quest for a more thorough understanding of foods and nutrition.

Books have the answers on how to gain optimum health, the Web does not. Books cannot be easily condensed into Web articles, and typically provide comprehensive coverage of the issues, or they refer to other books or studies that provide the information. In addition, books are typically written by competent and knowledgeable authors who provide good, proven advice.

Today's real need is not another low-carb, high-protein diet, or an end to global warming, which appears to be mainly caused by extensive deforestation efforts to clear space for cattle and feed crops. Rather, it is self-education about foods and nutrition.

Typically, people resort to doctors when they don't know what else to do. But by simply utilizing the Web/Internet, as well as the information that is contained in books that are available to most people, many health concerns can be thoroughly investigated, and the proper treatments determined, without seeing a physician.

The body can take a lot of punishment and abuse. It can survive both drought and famine. It can live on junk food for decades without showing many ill effects. But the body does not thrive on drought or famine or junk food. It thrives on life-giving plant foods. If optimum health is the goal, then a change in the diet is required.

None of us has to die of a disease caused by eating a bad diet, and none of us has to endure the many attendant complications and discomforts of a disease prior to death. And we won't, if we take care of our bodies by giving it the life-giving foods it needs.

It is our responsibility to take care of our bodies. It is not our doctor's, our spouse's, our friends' or the Government's. It is our responsibility. We should avoid foods that are harmful to health and eat foods that promote health and longevity. These are whole plant foods, replete with their life-giving properties. These are the foods that God and Nature intended for us to eat.

"But the foods which you eat from the abundant table of God give you strength and youth to your body, and you will never see disease. For the table of God fed Methuselah of old, and I tell you truly, if you live as he lived, then will the God of the living give you also long life upon the earth as was his." - Attributed to Jesus, The Essene Gospel of Peace, Book One.

• *Fruits and Vegetables*

Raw fruits and vegetables are eaten regularly on the raw vegan diet, for good reasons. They digest easily and efficiently because their enzymes have not been destroyed by heat. Enzymes have life force properties that Nature intended for us to receive, that support all bodily functions and contain the vitamins and nutrients the body needs for optimum health. (Note: enzymes are further discussed in the chapter on "The Dangers of Cooked Foods.")

Fruits and vegetables are best eaten when they are ripe. If eaten in their typical store-bought, un-ripened condition, stomachache or some other discomfort is likely. Also, extra energy is required to digest them, and this energy is taken from the energy reserves of the body when it could be used for other purposes such as healing and self-cleansing.

Fruits and vegetables sold at local food stores are typically shipped-in from distant locations, such as foreign countries, and purposely arrive in an un-ripened condition in order to retard spoilage and prolong shelf-life. To ripen store-bought fruits and vegetables, just set them on the counter tops at home until they are ripe; it usually takes several days, depending on the fruit or vegetable. For example, bananas are typically sold green or partly green in color, unless you happen by the fruit stand right before the bananas are replaced. Ripe bananas are speckled or streaked brown in color, which typically takes several days.

Cucumbers are ripe when they are easily flexed. Avocados are ripe when they yield to gentle pressure. Green chilies and jalapenos are ripe when they turn orange or red, do not eat them when they are green. Lemons, limes, oranges and pears are ripe when they are aromatic. Same for red and yellow peppers.

Some exceptions to this are apples (all varieties) and root vegetables (e.g., carrots, beets, turnips, radishes, potatoes, onions, garlic, etc.). Apples and root vegetables do not ripen to any significant extent after they are picked.

Fruits are nutritious and stimulating, and have many healing qualities. They act to cleanse and energize the cells of the body. I consider fruits to be the ideal food for humankind.

"Fruits alone, even of but one kind, not only heal but nourish perfectly the human body, eliminating entirely the possibility of disease." - Arnold Ehret, Mucusless Diet Healing System.

Some people will not eat fruit because the last time they did, it caused them too much discomfort. Most likely, it was because the fruit was eaten in an un-ripened condition, or else it was combined improperly with other foods. For example, when dates or figs are eaten with pineapple, the result may be a stomachache, because sweet fruit (dates and figs) should not be eaten with acid fruit (pineapple). See the chapter on "Proper Food Combinations."

The importance of eating fruit on the raw vegan diet cannot be overemphasized, and will be discussed further in this book.

Fatty fruits include avocados and olives. They contain healthy unsaturated fat. Some nutritional experts consider avocado a Superfood, although it is not classified as such. Superfoods have super high-density nutritional value (see subsection on Superfoods). The avocado contains a substantial amount of monounsaturated fats, phytosterols and antioxidants like vitamin E, vitamin C, and carotenoids. It is also high in beta-sitosterol (95 mg per medium-sized avocado) which is known to assist in relieving prostate disorders, such as benign prostatic hyperplasia (BPH).

Plain avocado can be used like butter on raw vegetables such as cabbage, broccoli, cucumber, cauliflower, carrots, asparagus, green onions, tomatoes, chili peppers and celery - with great results. Or, you can make an avocado-based dipping sauce, such as the one described below. But it's mainly fat, so use avocado in moderation.

The vegetables that have the most tightly compacted layers are some of the most nutritious. They include red and green cabbage, leeks, broccoli, bok choy, green onions, lettuce and celery.

Carrots are high in beta-carotene which is converted to vitamin A in the body. The word "carotene" is derived from the Latin word for carrot, "carota." Nutritional expert N.W. Walker in his books (see Bibliography), states that raw carrots have all the elements and vitamins that are required by the human body. It could just be that the lowly carrot is capable of making up for many of the nutritional deficiencies in the world today.

Carrots are non-starchy vegetables (see the chapter on "Proper Food Combinations").

Red beets are good for the blood. They lower blood pressure. They improve athletic performance. They are one of the highest of oxygenating foods. Marathon runners are partial to them because they increase their endurance. After consuming red beets, it takes less energy to run a race. This makes red beets important for elderly health, since studies have shown that there is a decline in maximal oxygen consumption with age. In addition, red beets have a high acid-binding rating (see Berg's Tables in the Appendix).

I haven't forgotten about leafy greens, which are one of the most important foods we can eat on the raw vegan diet. I consider them their own food group as will be discussed soon.

A Vegetable Dipping Sauce

A meal that makes you sit straight up in a chair is a tasty meal. Raw plant foods do not have to be boring, bland affairs. They can be tasty meals, and, for effective digestion, the mouth should water before and during a meal.

There are plenty of nutritious raw plant food recipes in well-thought-out raw food recipe books, such as Kristina Carrillo-Bucaram's book, The Fully Raw Diet.

I would avoid using raw food recipes on the Web, since they often combine fruits and vegetables improperly. No one needs to turn a meal into a gastronomic catastrophe. Meals should be tasty, but they should go easy on the stomach.

The following dipping sauce makes all vegetables and greens more palatable. While intended for those just starting out on a whole plant food diet, it can be used with great success also by experienced raw food eaters. It is the only recipe in this book.

How to Make the Sauce:

• Prepare several large avocados, sans skins, in a large bowl or container.
• Blend (using a blender) a few large carrots and/or red beets in water, and then add them to the avocados.
• Blend 5 lemons, 5 garlic cloves, and 1 skinned red or yellow onion (or 2 bunches of green onions) in water, and add to the mixture.
• Add unrefined, natural sea salt to taste (for the benefits of using natural sea salt, see the chapter on "The Good and Bad About Salt").

The sauce has six important tastes to stimulate the corresponding six groups of taste buds – sour (lemons), spicy (garlic), bitter (onions), fat (avocado), sweet (all vegetables contain natural sugars) and salty. It makes rainbow kale or broccoli sprouts a complete meal, and enhances the taste of all other vegetables.

No short cuts! A mistake that raw food eaters sometimes make is taking short cuts. If lemon or lime juice from 100% concentrate is used in the above dipping sauce recipe, we are adding cooked foods because juice from 100% concentrate is a pasteurized, processed food product. If you are faithful to the raw vegan diet, you will reap the full benefits of the diet.

No fruit or vegetable is intrinsically better than another. Each may be preferred, or not, depending on a person's nutritional needs and personal preferences. We all have grown to like certain fruits or vegetables better than others, and we all have slightly different nutritional needs. The only way to learn what fruits and vegetables are best for us, is to eat a variety of them in their ripened states, and, if not by themselves in mono meals, then ensuring that they are eaten properly combined with other foods.

David Wolfe states in one of his books that there are so many edible fruits and vegetables in the world that if you tried a new kind every day of your life, you would never live long enough to try them all. So, what is stopping us from trying the 40-50 varieties of fruits and vegetables that are in our local food stores? It's the only way to know whether they work for us nutritionally and otherwise.

Grains and Legumes

Technically speaking, grains are seeds of grasses. However, they are commonly considered to be vegetables. Grains include wheat, corn, oats, barley, rye, millet, and rice. Grain products include refined flour products, such as white bread, cereal, white and brown rice and pasta.

Most grains are starchy foods. For that reason, I no longer eat grains, nor do I advise their use on the raw vegan diet. If you eat grains, they should be kept to a minimum part of the diet. Many nutritionists believe that eating these foods leads to constipation and then to disease. More about this is provided in the chapter on "The Dangers of Starchy Foods."

Legumes include peas, beans, peanuts and lentils. Legumes are commonly considered to be vegetables. Like grains, they are starchy foods, and for that reason I no longer eat them, nor do I advise their use on the raw vegan diet.

● *Greens (Leafy Green Vegetables)*

Leafy greens are commonly considered vegetables, but I agree with Victoria Boutenko in her book, *Green for Life*, that greens should be their own food group. Greens are the only foods that combine well with all other foods, including other greens. You can't say that about many fruits and vegetables or nuts and seeds.

Leafy greens include spinach, arugula, chard, kale (several varieties), mustard greens, collard greens, turnip greens, parsley, cilantro, lettuce (several varieties), celery greens and dandelion.

A good way to add greens to our diet is to drink green smoothies. They provide the health benefits of fruits and greens in a single meal. Try apricots, bananas, lemons, mangos (in season) with kale, spinach, romaine lettuce, or chard. Watch the way you combine fruits to ensure adherence to the food combination laws, which are discussed in the chapter on "Proper Food Combinations." You should rotate the greens every week or so to avoid alkaloid buildup, which is caused when too much of one kind of greens are eaten.

The chlorophyll in greens strengthens the immune system, helps to detoxify the body and improves digestion. Chlorophyll is rich in antioxidants, minerals, vitamins and readily assimilated enzymes. The chlorophyll in green plants is what converts sunlight into chemical energy, and this energy is made available to us when we eat greens.

Eating a variety of greens ensures that we receive all the amino acids we need in our diets. In his book, *The China Study,* T. Colin Campbell states that plant protein is the healthiest type of protein because it allows for slow but steady synthesis of the proteins.

"Greens are the primary food group that matches human nutritional needs most completely…Chlorophyll is liquefied sun energy. Consuming as much chlorophyll as possible is like bathing our inner organs in sunshine." - Victoria Boutenko, Green for Life.

Cilantro is high in potassium and vitamins A, B, C and K and has antifungal, antioxidant and antibacterial properties.

Women should eat more greens. It is known that menstruation difficulties or pains find their solution in eating greens. The importance of eating greens cannot be overemphasized, for the simple reason that few things in life are more important for health.

Store-bought arugula (shipped-in from elsewhere, not locally) is much milder than the arugula I get from my local Community Supported Agriculture (CSA) farm. The CSA arugula is noticeably spicier (more peppery), like mild chili peppers. What does this difference in taste mean? Studies have shown that foods grown locally and harvested recently are superior nutritionally to store-bought foods. You can taste the difference. The studies show that fruits and vegetables lose vitamins while in storage and transit. Lettuce loses about 50% of its key nutrients. For Web articles about this, e.g., search on "home grown vs. store bought produce."

The cost difference between organic and conventionally grown produce is typically only a matter of nickels and dimes, rather than dollars as it used to be. In my opinion, the advantages of organic foods far outweigh any small cost differential.

The Importance of Organic Foods

Federal regulations in the US stipulate that organic foods cannot be grown with synthetic (man-made) fertilizers, synthetic pesticides or sewage sludge. As such, organic foods do not contain harmful or potentially toxic substances. These regulations were a long time in coming.

Organic foods are not irradiated[2], and they are not GMO-modified (i.e., Genetically Modified Organisms). Organic produce will typically have the "USDA Organic" label, but may have the "CCOF (California Certified Organic Farmers) Organic" label which is somewhat less restrictive than the "USDA Organic" label. Other organizations are also USDA certified, such as Oregon Tilth, which uses the "Oregon Tilth Certified Organic" (OTCO) label.

There are now more certified organic growers/farmers in this country than ever before. Accordingly, prices have gone down for organic foods.

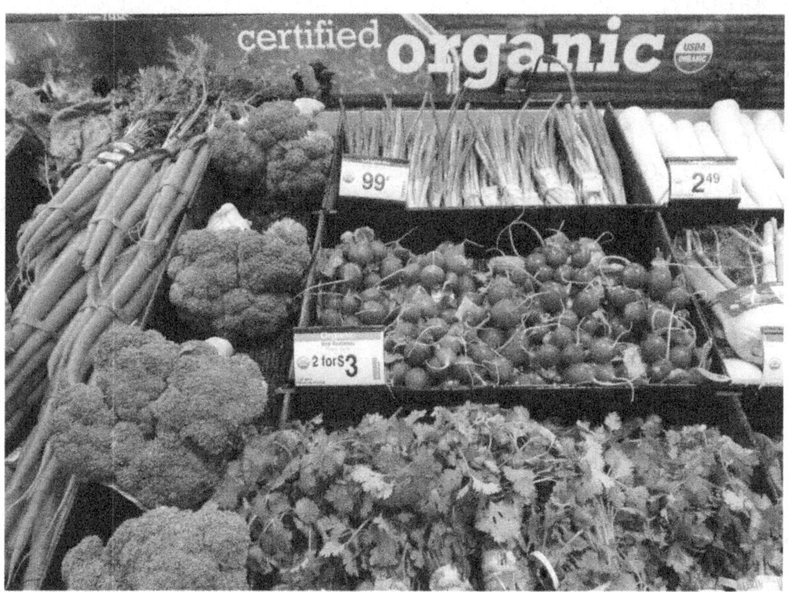

We can buy non-organic bananas, lemons, limes, pineapples, avocados, onions and garlic because they require less pesticides in their cultivation, so they should have less pesticide residues on them. Also, we don't usually eat the skins of these foods. In addition, they are non-GMO crops (see the chapter on "GMO Crops").

---

[2] Dr. Edward Howell states in his book, Enzyme Nutrition, that the use of radiation to preserve foods results in the wholesale destruction of all the enzymes and vital properties contained in the foods.

Pesticides

Pesticides are poisons that are sprayed on conventionally-grown plant foods in order to kill pests that attack the crops. USDA tests have shown that pesticide contamination levels on plant foods can vary depending on the crop and where it is grown.

If pesticides can kill other life forms, then they may also be injurious to human life. Studies have shown that pesticides are indeed injurious to human health. The dangers of pesticides are adequately covered on the Web, and in the books listed in the Bibliography.

Lists of fruits and vegetables that have the least and the most pesticides on them are provided on the Web. Two of these lists, the "Clean 15" and the "Dirty Dozen", are provided in Appendix II. However, a comment about these lists is in order. Not all fruits and vegetables are included in these lists. Also, the lists may not be completely reliable. For example, cabbage, which is one of my favorite vegetables, is listed in the "Clean 15" list, indicating that I can purchase it conventionally grown and do not have to buy it "organic."

However, according to David Wolfe's book, *The Sunfood Diet Success System*, large amounts of pesticides are used on non-organic cabbage. I searched the Web to confirm this but could not find the information of Wolfe's book on the Web. I wanted to be sure, so I ate non-organic white/green cabbage for a week. Small red, itchy sores erupted on my skin, and I'm not allergic to cabbage. I have the same reaction whenever I eat non-organic foods that have high pesticide residues. While this is not conclusive or scientific proof, it leads me to believe that cabbage should not be listed on the "Clean 15" list.

• *Nuts and Seeds*

To get our daily complement of saturated fats, nuts and seeds may be eaten. Nuts come from trees. The peanut, which is not really a nut but a legume, grows in the ground.

Nuts and seeds contain vitamins, minerals and folic acid which are needed by the body. However, many of the commercially available nuts and seeds are refined and processed foods that should not be eaten on the diet. They include the many roasted and salted varieties. The life force properties of these foods have been destroyed by heat. A roasted or pasteurized nut or seed planted in the ground will not grow.

I used to buy "raw almonds" from the local food stores. The labels clearly state "Raw Almonds." However, I learned that almonds are required by law (such as California State law) to be steam-pasteurized. The same goes for hazelnuts (filberts). Therefore, if we buy "raw" almonds or hazelnuts purchased from local food stores, the chances are we are buying pasteurized nuts with their enzymes destroyed. Pasteurized nuts have some nutritional value but they do not have the life force properties of raw plant foods, and should therefore be avoided on the diet.

Nuts and seeds easily absorb pesticides. Many are imported from distant countries, such as Africa, where food products may not be properly monitored or controlled for pesticide residues. Per the Web, peanuts, pistachios and cashews have the worst pesticide residues. Therefore, to minimize pesticides in your diet, buy raw, "organic" nuts and seeds. If you cannot find them at local food stores, they can be purchased from websites.

Nuts and seeds combine well with themselves and with most vegetables. Fatty nuts (like pecans) combine well with sweet fruits.

FAT VS PROTEIN CONTENT OF NUTS AND SEEDS (FAT / PROTEIN)

Almonds	2/1
Brazil Nuts	4/1
Cashews	2/1

Hazelnuts	4/1
Pecans	10/1
Pistachios	2/1
Walnuts	4/1
Pumpkin Seeds	1.5/1
Sunflower Seeds	3/1

As seen above, nuts and seeds are fat-dominant foods, not protein-dominant foods. David Wolfe, in *The Sunfood Diet Success System*, agrees. However, this is not reflected in many articles on the Web which claim that nuts and seeds are protein-dominant foods. More on this in the chapter on "Proper Food Combinations."

Sprouting

I believe that everyone on the raw vegan diet should learn how to sprout foods. It puts you in the driver's seat and gives you complete control over what you eat.

Sprouts are the initial forms of plants after they germinate from seeds. When a seed germinates, its life force is at a peak level. Eating sprouts is highly recommended for their abundant supply of enzymes and nutrients. Fully sprouted seeds, such as broccoli sprouts, can be purchased from whole food stores. Whether purchased or home-grown, sprouts should be included in the raw vegan diet on a frequent basis.

Soaking raw nuts and seeds in water causes them to sprout. Some exceptions to this, however, are pecans, walnuts and Brazil nuts.

Basically, here's how to sprout nuts and seeds at home. Add raw (unpasteurized) nuts or seeds to a quart jar to about 1/2 full because they will expand when soaked, then fill with water and let them soak overnight. In the morning, drain the water and let them dry sufficiently. You can dry them at home in the kitchen, in the sun or you can use a dehydrator at about 115° F. Drying times can be several days or more. When they are thoroughly dry, then eat them and benefit from their abundant life force.

When I began sprouting, I read sprouting books, purchased the seeds, quart jars and wicker baskets, and learned the proper techniques. You can best learn how to grow your own sprouts at home by reading Dr. Ann Wigmore's book, *The Sprouting Book*, and Steve ("Sproutman") Meyerowitz's book, *Sprouts, The Miracle Food*.

Sprouting is a survival tactic that may be useful someday. The basics required are only seeds, water, air and a little sunshine. A person could live a long time on nothing but sprouts.

Sprouting can be messy and clutter up the kitchen, but that can be avoided or minimized by the sprouting method used. There are now some very inventive and easy to use DIY kits available on the Web for sprouting at home. In any case, the remarkable life force in sprouts outweighs any minor inconveniences.

• *Sea Vegetables*

"The composition of the human body and the composition of seven gallons of sea water are the same. In view of this fact, it would seem practical to turn to the sea in order to supply the nutrient needs of the body." - Dr. D. C. Jarvis, <u>Folk Medicine</u>.

Sea vegetables are important adjuncts to land vegetables in the raw vegan diet. As mentioned previously, the topsoil worldwide is minerally deficient. Sea vegetables obtain their minerals from the ocean, which is a mineral-rich environment and practically unaffected by topsoil mineral deficiency.

Sea vegetables, including kelp and dulse, are our main source of iodine. Sea vegetables are also high in potassium. Both of these minerals are often lacking in today's land-grown crops. Iodine is needed for the proper functioning of the thyroid gland and potassium is needed for the proper functioning of the nervous system.

While natural sea salt contains iodine from the sea, it provides less of what we need daily. Nutritional experts such as Dr. D. C. Jarvis, recommend taking 1/4 to 1/2 teaspoons of kelp or dulse per day to meet the daily iodine requirement.

"There is a definite relationship between the amount of energy you have and your iodine intake." - Dr. D. C. Jarvis, <u>Folk Medicine</u>.

According to Dr. Bernard Jensen in his book, *Guide to Diet and Detoxification*, dulse may be the best source of iodine because it contains more manganese which assists in the absorption of iodine in the body. Kelp and dulse are available in powder, tablet and liquid form.

When I was macrobiotic years ago, I ate brown rice balls with nori, a sea vegetable. When I switched to a vegetarian diet with fish, I stopped eating nori. I now eat sea vegetables almost daily and have experienced their benefits.

However, do not discount the possibility that your tastes and food choices will change with time on the raw vegan diet.

• *Superfoods*

Superfoods are the foods of the future in the sense that many people are not familiar with them. David Wolfe in his book, *Superfoods*, defines them as: "plant foods with super high-density nutritional value."

In my opinion, Superfoods should be added cautiously to the diet because of their potency and unique characteristics. The road to Superfoods turns into some very exciting country, but go slow, there are some hazards.

I recommend adding only one Superfood at a time to the diet, so that each may be tested to see what they do for you, or against you. That way you avoid the pitfalls of eating Superfoods together and possibly violating food combination laws, and also, you'll be better able to utilize the knowledge gained about each Superfood when it is advantageous for you to do so.

The following Superfoods are discussed herein.

● Aloe Vera

● Spirulina

● Hemp Seed

● Goji Berries

● Bee Products

● Cacao Beans

● Maca

● Coconut

There are more Superfoods than those listed, but those discussed are the most commonly eaten on the raw vegan diet. For more Superfood information, see David Wolfe's book, *Superfoods*.

Aloe Vera

Aloe Vera is a medium-sized, green and firm-leaf plant with leaves consisting of a gelatinous interior surrounded by a skin with thorns on the edges of the leaves. It is rich in antioxidants, amino acids and enzymes that help cleanse the body of toxins. It is well known to have curative powers for healing cuts and burns. You don't have to de-skin the leaves or cut off the thorns; each leaf can be eaten raw. Aloe Vera, like chayote, has very little aroma until it is cut into.

Like the palm tree, it grows without much assistance in sunny climates. To eat Aloe Vera, cut off the lower leaves which are the first to droop and die. If the leaves are stored in the refrigerator, they last for weeks. After a few days of storage, the thorns are soft enough to eat, so you don't have to remove them.

Eating more than a small amount of Aloe Vera leaf per day may cause gas or other complications. Aloe Vera is a very effective bowel cleanser.

Spirulina

Spirulina is a blue-green fresh water algae. It is typically grown in lakes. It is lauded for its amazing health benefits. It is high in protein, and contains antioxidants, B-complex vitamins, beta-carotene, vitamin E, manganese, zinc, copper, iron, selenium, and gamma linolenic acid. It is one of the few plant sources of the DHA/EPA and ALA omega-3 fatty acids, the other being chlorella.

Spirulina is about 50% protein by weight, making it one of the highest protein plant foods available. On the raw vegan diet, it is easy to get all the protein you need from leafy greens and vegetables, but if you're worried about not getting enough protein, then add spirulina to your next meal. However, watch how you combine it with other foods.

Spirulina is typically sold in powdered form which is easily added to anything.

Despite its many benefits, I have found that spirulina causes very foul-smelling gas. Spirulina is a form of bacteria, of the phylum Cyanobacteria. When it gets into the intestines it can cause friendly bacteria to proliferate to an extent that causes excess gas.

Chlorella, also considered a superfood, is similar to spirulina and also causes smelly gas, at least for me. For that reason, I no longer use these products.

Hemp Seed

Hemp Seed is said to be the most nutritious seed in the world. It contains all the essential amino acids and fatty acids that are required for human life. It is high in protein (but not as much as spirulina – see table below), antioxidants, iron, zinc, carotene, phytosterols, vitamins and enzymes. Hemp seeds have an ideal ratio of omega 6 to omega 3 fatty acids, and because of this they are preferred over flaxseeds and chia seeds for omega 3.

When I first tried hemp seeds, I was surprised that they were not hard seeds like many other seeds. They are soft seeds and have a mild, nutty, or grain-like flavor.

Goji Berries

Goji berries, which are native to China, are bright-red berries that grow on shrubs. They are high in antioxidants and nutrients. They make an excellent snack food when eaten by themselves. However, when combined with other foods, except for greens, the combinations should adhere to the food combination laws (see chapter on Proper Food Combinations).

Contrary to articles on the Web which indicate that goji berries combine well with sweet fruit, such as raisons, and also with protein foods, such as nuts, seeds and hemp seed, as in trail mix, I discovered it was not the case. Such food combinations cause stomachaches indicative of not adhering to the laws of nature that include the rules of proper food combining.

Almost all goji berries sold on the market today are of the dried fruit kind. They look, feel and taste like raisins. But unlike raisins, which are sweet fruit, goji berries, in my opinion, are acid or sub-acid fruit. They combine well with pineapple, cherries and raspberries, but do not combine well with sweet fruit, such as figs or grapes, or with protein foods, such as nuts and seeds.

Goji berries have the peculiar distinction of being adaptogens, which are substances that exert a normalizing effect on bodily processes. Ginseng is a well-known example.

I first purchased goji berries from local whole foods stores, but later found better prices on the Web.

Bee Products[3]

Bee product superfoods include honey, bee pollen and royal jelly. Another bee product, honeycomb, is not considered a superfood.

Honey is made by bees from the nectar of flowers and plants that bees visit when pollenating them. Raw honey contains many minerals, amino acids and enzymes.

Most of the honey consumed today is refined honey, which is pasteurized so its enzymes have been destroyed. If the label does not say "raw," then it is refined and processed honey.

Dr. D. C. Jarvis in his book, *Arthritis and Folk Medicine*, states that the nutritional value of foods is improved by the ability of honey to extract from the foods what the body needs. He also states that it has been the experience of generations of Vermonters that beekeepers do not have kidney trouble, and do not develop cancer or paralysis.

David Wolfe in his book, *Superfoods*, states that bee pollen is the most complete Superfood there is. Royal jelly, another bee

---

[3] Bee products are often contested as not being raw vegan food since they come from bees, which are animals. However, there are many nutritionists, among them Ann Wigmore, Norman W. Walker, Herbert M. Shelton and David Wolf, who advocate including bee products in the raw vegan diet. In my opinion, this issue is, in the overall picture of things, a minor point of contestability, especially when the health benefits of bee products are considered. In any case, each of us must decide how we stand on this issue. Like any other types of food, if bee products do not work for you, then they should be avoided.

product, is what bees feed to the larvae in the hive. It is also highly nutritious.

Unfortunately, the worldwide population of bees is declining. The on-going extinction is blamed on the widespread use of pesticides on crops. This has the potential of adversely affecting all of us. If it is not turned around soon, it will have dire consequences for the pollination of plants, which means the production of fruits and all other plants that require pollination for their reproduction. This tragedy is documented in Horst Kornberger's book, *Global Hive: Bee Crisis and Compassionate Ecology*. The Web adequately covers this issue. It is also covered in some DVDs that are available on the subject.

Organic, raw, unfiltered honey has not been adulterated in any way and is the best honey to eat for health benefits. You can squeeze honey on salads, add unrefined sea salt and some water, and it tastes like French dressing. Or add it to apple cider vinegar to make a cure all drink that has been used for centuries in the US to cure many human ailments (see the last section of this chapter).

Cacao Beans

Cacao beans are not really beans (legumes) but the seeds of the cacao tree.

Cacao beans are very high in antioxidants and nutrients. Crushed cacao beans are called cacao nibs. Cacao nibs have been dried and fermented but are apparently the least processed of the available forms of chocolate. If you want to try a more natural form chocolate, then cacao nibs are the product to buy. Cacao nibs are crunchy and have a slightly bitter taste. Soaking cacao nibs in water makes them softer and easier to chew.

There are two powdered forms of the cacao bean: 1) cacao powder and 2) cocoa powder. They are similar but not the same thing. They taste the same, but taste is often deceiving. Both cacao powder and cocoa powder are refined and processed foods, but cacao powder is the least refined form. Cacao powder is made by cold-pressing unroasted cacao beans. It is claimed that the cold-pressing process does not destroy any of the bean's enzymes and nutrients. Cocoa powder is made by roasting the cacao beans.

A useful yardstick of food value is Oxygen Radical Absorbance Capacity (ORAC), which is an antioxidant rating that was used by the USDA until 2012. It is still used as a comparative basis for antioxidant capacity. Per the Web, the ORAC value of raw cacao powder is 95,500, which is the highest rating of all forms of chocolate. The ORAC value of roasted cocoa powder is 26,000. More about ORAC in the chapter on "Antioxidants."

Everyone likes chocolate, but have you tried the genuine article, cacao nibs?

Maca

Maca, like goji berries, is also an adaptogen. Maca is known to increase energy levels and enhance libido. Some claim that it is an aphrodisiac. It is typically sold in powdered form, which is easily added to anything.

Maca has a butterscotch color and a mild, butterscotch flavor. When I first tried it, I combined it with spirulina in my vegetable dipping sauce. This resulted in violating a food combination law and caused me to have a big stomachache. Maca is a starchy food, whereas spirulina is a protein food. Starchy foods and protein foods should not be eaten together (see the chapter on "Proper Food Combinations"). However, when properly combined with other foods, Maca adds real gusto to life. When I combined it properly, I was impressed by the increase in energy I experienced.

Maca is also available in a near starch-free powder, called Gelatinized Maca, but the product undergoes additional refining and does not have the life force properties of regular Maca.

In my opinion, Maca is a very powerful Superfood. We don't understand all of its benefits, but it should be used moderately.

Maca is 32% starch (see the chapter on "Proper Food Combinations"). It is, therefore, a starchy food. I no longer eat Maca because I no longer eat starchy foods (see the chapter on "The Dangers of Starchy Foods").

Coconut

Coconut provides health benefits, such as protecting against heart disease and stroke, and has the capability to neutralize or eradicate Candida and other pathogenic microorganisms. It is tasty by itself or when combined with chocolate (cacao beans), and it also makes a great addition to green smoothies.

Coconut is about one-third saturated fat. The saturated fat in coconut is a healthy saturated fat, which is different from the saturated fat found in animal products. The saturated fat in coconut is a medium-chain fatty acid that is easily assimilated by the body. The saturated fat in animal products is a long-chain fatty acid that is difficult to assimilate by the body. Coconut does not contribute to blood cholesterol levels as opposed to the long-chain fatty acids that are found in animal products.[4]

To open a coconut, the recommended approach is to wrap it in a towel and hit it with a hammer. I use a plastic grocery bag instead of a towel for easier clean up. The Web may be useful here. It has YouTube videos on how to open and peel coconuts. You can drop them on the floor to crack them open. Then, pry the shell apart with a large knife, and separate the meat from the shell using a knife or other tool. The meat can be frozen for later use.

The protein content of selected raw plant foods is given below, compiled from books in the Bibliography and from Web articles.

---

[4] Coconut oil, the kind typically sold in bottles, is a fractionated oil that is known to raise cholesterol levels in people, per Victoria Boutenko's book, <u>Raw & Beyond</u>. Fractionated oils also include other so-called "healthy" oils, such as olive oil and avocado oil. It is best to stay away from oils.

Some may find it useful for ensuring adherence to the food combination laws, and it should dampen the fears of those who are worried about not getting enough protein on the raw vegan diet.

PROTEIN CONTENT OF RAW PLANT FOODS

Spirulina	50%
Hemp Seeds	30%
Pumpkin Seeds	28%
Pistachios	20%
Sesame Seeds	20%
Cacao Beans	20%
Flaxseeds	20%
Chia Seeds	14%
Sunflower Seeds	11%

Not everyone has the same proclivity, or liking, for foods, or the same nutritional requirements. But the body requires similar things for health and wellness, and we are all very much alike in numerous ways, having the same basic needs, the same general physiology, the same susceptibility to biological disharmony, the same susceptibility to many illnesses, and we share many of the same stresses, worries and fears that can influence our state of health. Nutritionists, whose voices have not been heard as much as those of ordinary diet proponents, have been telling us for years that ill health and diseases of all types spring most often from one common source, namely, poor dietary practices.

The best diet is the one that meets the energy and nutrient needs of the body and produces the least negative effects, such as toxicity, acidity and constipation. For most people, it means a diet consisting of a large volume of fresh, raw fruits and vegetables to meet the body's nutrient needs, and enough concentrated foods, such as nuts and seeds, to meet the body's energy needs.

"If you diligently heed the voice of the Lord your God and do what is right in His sight, give ear to His commandments and keep all His statutes, I will put none of the diseases on you which I have brought on the Egyptians." - Ex. 15:26.

The Importance of Apple Cider Vinegar and Honey

Apple cider vinegar (not the white distilled or wine vinegars) is known to assist in the digestion of foods. As explained in Victoria Boutenko's book, *Green for Life*, hydrochloric acid production in the stomach decreases after age 40. A low stomach acid condition is blamed for various nutritional deficiencies due to the inability of the body to adequately digest foods and absorb nutrients. It is also blamed for the greying of hair. Nutritional experts claim that supplementing the diet with apple cider vinegar helps to restore stomach acid to its proper levels.

Dr. N.W. Walker in his book Fresh Vegetable and Fruit Juices, states that apple cider vinegar contains malic acid, which is absent in white distilled and wine vinegars. Malic acid is beneficial to the body. All vinegars, including apple cider vinegar, are acidic, but as explained in his book, diluted apple cider vinegar is alkalizing to the body. In addition, malic acid can be stored in the body as glycogen for future use, and is known to promote healthy blood vessels, veins and arteries, and aid in coagulating the blood in establishing a normal menstrual flow.

Apple cider vinegar is made by fermenting crushed apples, which makes it different from other vinegars such as white or wine vinegars which are made by fermenting alcohol. Apple cider vinegar has the highest pH of any vinegar, 3.3 to 3.5. Other vinegars have a pH of around 2.4 making then more acidic. The lower the pH, the more acidic is the solution (pH is a logarithmic scale).

GMO Crops

Currently, according to the Web, there are ten (10) genetically modified food crops commercially available. They are listed below with the year they became commercially available. Other crops have been genetically modified as well, but they are either no longer commercially available because they were withdrawn from the market due to unfavorable reception, or they are in the process of being patented.

Soybeans, 1995

Squash, 1995

Corn (field and sweet), 1996[5]

Cotton, 1996

Papaya, 1997

Canola (rapeseed), 1999

Alfalfa, 2006

Sugar beets, 2006

Potatoes, 2016

Apples, 2017

All the above foods are for human consumption (cottonseed oil is often used in food products), and some are also used for livestock feed.

---

[5] However, according to a 2014 EWG article, most corn on the cob sweet corn has not been genetically engineered, but corn-based sweeteners, starches and oils used in processed foods are GMO.

Upwards of 75% of the refined and processed foods on supermarket shelves contain GMO products. GMO sweet corn and sugar beets are widely used in refined and processed foods as "sugar" or high-fructose corn syrup (HFCS). GMO soybeans are widely used as soy in many refined and processed foods. Soy is found in almost all baked goods and imitation dairy products, and also in alternative meat products such as veggie burgers. Soy derivatives include hydrolyzed plant protein (HPP), hydrolyzed soy protein (HSP) and/or hydrolyzed vegetable protein (HVP), which are added to a wide range of refined and processed foods, including soda, chips, salad dressings and soups.

GMO (Genetically Modified Organism) refers to a plant or animal (e.g., a fish) that is artificially created by inserting genes from one species into the DNA of another species. GE (Genetically Engineered) is another term used for genetically-altered foods.

Many GMO creations have been, and are now being, patented and released into our environment and food supply, and there seems to be no end in sight. Of course, if we buy all our foods "organic", that is, having the proper "Organic" label on them, then we should not have to worry about GMO foods, at least not for the present. This was covered in the last chapter under the section, "The Importance of Organic Foods."

One of the reasons for developing GMO crops was to make them more pesticide- and herbicide-resistant so they could tolerate lethal herbicides and pesticides that non-GMO crops cannot tolerate.

There are two main health concerns associated with consuming GMO crops. First, the highly poisonous pesticides and herbicides that are used on these crops may leave high residues on the crops or they may seep into the crops themselves. We know that the pesticides and herbicides used on non-GMO crops leave residues and can seep into the crops.

The second danger is the risk to human health of the Bt (Bacillus thuringiensis) toxin, which is genetically inserted into the DNA of the crop species. The cells of the species that are modified are genetically engineered to include the Bt toxin in order to kill the pests that feed on the crops. The toxin acts as a delayed-action bomb that goes off when pests eat the crops. Crops that have been modified to take the Bt toxin include corn, cotton, and soybeans.

The flurry of reports that were the rage of the 1990s and early 2000s about the health hazards of GMO foods are no longer in the news. The reports have become much less frequent, replaced by carefully-worded reports and articles that are sponsored by food industry advocates of the food industry, that support the continued use of GMO crops. The principal pro-GMO argument is that GMO crops resist many food viruses and pests, thus making them more available to more people. However, these reports and articles, many of which are on the Web, fail to adequately address, for many people, the earlier-identified dangers of consuming these foods. As a result of these developments, public attention as a whole has shifted away from the dangers of GMOs to other concerns.

There is a scarcity of scientific studies on humans to justify the health risks that are associated with the above-described dangers. But there have been numerous reports showing that human health is adversely affected by these crops. These reports are not limited to the adverse health effects on farm workers who spray the pesticides and herbicides on the crops, but include people who eat the GMO crops.

One of the difficulties in assessing studies done on the human health effects of GMO crops is the fact the evaluation of GE herbicide-resistant crops is conducted by USDA, their evaluation when the crops can be consumed by people is conducted by FDA, while the herbicides are assessed by EPA when there are new potential exposures.[6]

---

[6] 2016 NCBI report on the Web, entitled, "Human Health Effects of Genetically Engineered Crops."

However, it stands to reason that if the strong pesticides and herbicides that are sprayed on GMO crops adversely affect the health of GMO farm workers, then the same poisons may adversely affect the health of people who consume the GMO crops. And, if eating GMO crops that have the Bt toxin kills insects, then eating the crops may adversely affect human health in some way.

At the time of this writing, there are no requirements to label GMO food "GMO" or "GE" or anything else to alert consumers of what they are buying. This is despite opinion polls that show that up to 90 percent of Americans want GMO foods labeled.

"Is there any intelligent being who is so naïve as to assume that the poisons will be less devastating to the human body, with its endlessly more intricate and delicate living mechanism?" - Dr. Lars-Eric Essen.

On the raw vegan diet, only raw, natural foods are consumed. Therefore, if you are on the diet you should not worry about consuming GMO foods, unless you buy non-organic produce. In that case, you should ensure that the produce is not a GMO food by checking the list above or an updated list as time goes by. If any of the foods you buy are purchased non-organic, that is, not having a "USDA Organic" "CCOF Organic" or OTCO label on them (as discussed previously), then they are likely to be GMO foods.

Not all varieties of foods that are listed above have been genetically modified, at least not as yet. For example, there are over a hundred varieties of apples, one of my favorite foods, but only one variety, Artic apples, has been genetically modified as of this writing according to the Web.

Potatoes that are genetically modified include the White Russet potatoes which are used worldwide in fast-food restaurants for fries.

"The huge jump in childhood food allergies in the US is in the news often, but most reports fail to consider a link to a recent radical change in America's diet. Beginning in 1996, bacteria, virus and other genes have been artificially inserted to the DNA of soy, corn, cottonseed and canola plants. These unlabeled genetically modified (GM) foods carry a risk of triggering life-threatening allergic reactions, and evidence collected over the past decade now suggests that they are contributing to higher allergy rates." - Jeffery M. Smith, from a Web article.

It would seem that the wide-spread consumption of GMO crops in our society is the population study, or test, that these crops will have to see what happens to human health as a result of eating them. It also appears that everyone who consumes GMO crops is an individual test case. It appears that we are all guinea pigs in a gigantic experiment, and no one knows for sure what the outcome will be. That is not a good way to conduct a scientific study on human heath, nor is it good policy!

In addition to the human health dangers, GMO crops contaminate non-GE counterparts, for example corn. Cross-pollination has led to the widespread contamination of non-GMO corn crops. Controlling the spread of GE contamination has proven to be all but impossible. Since this threat is so real and prevalent, it is best to restrict one's diet to food types that have not been genetically engineered.

Two popular DVDs have explored and documented the dangers of GMO crops, Genetic Roulette and The GMO Trilogy. Both are by Jeffery M. Smith, who authored the books Seeds of Deception and Genetic Roulette that the movies are based on.

Although the controversy about the health hazards of eating GMO crops seems to have faded into the past, we need to keep vigilant on what is going on in the food industry if we wish to improve and maintain our health, especially since so much health information today is being controlled by vested interests that care much more about their profit than our health.

The Dangers of Cooked Foods

"If you eat living food, the same will quicken you, but if you kill your food the dead food will kill you also. For life comes only from life, and from death always comes death." - Attributed to Jesus, <u>The Essene Gospel of Peace, Book One</u>.

Nutritional experts have stressed for years that cooked foods are harmful to human health, and that the cooking of foods done at home and in restaurants, and in the food factories that manufacture canned, bottled and jarred foods, reduces the food value of the foods by altering their chemical properties and destroying important food constituents such as enzymes and nutrients, which also includes vitamins. They have also been telling us that cooked foods of almost any kind create acidity in the body. It is now known that cooking and the refining and processing of foods are responsible for the development of many of the sicknesses and diseases that plague humankind.

As stated previously, Americans eat more cooked food than any people on earth, and spend more money on doctor bills and healthcare than any people on earth. It appears to be more than a coincidence.

The fast food franchises, as well as other eating establishments, grill, fry, bake, and steam-heat their foods, or use dehydrated foods that have already been refined and processed using these methods. It has been known for years that these methods destroy important food components such as enzymes, vitamins and other nutrients, and also alter the chemical properties of the foods.

Robert Morse in his book, *The Detox Miracle Sourcebook*, explains how cooking dramatically decreases the molecular energy of foods, since heat affects the electrons of the food molecules and alters their molecular structure. However, when we eat raw foods, their high electromagnetic energy is transferred to the body and its cells.

Dr. N. W. Walker in many of his books, such as *Colon Health* and *Become Younger*, tells us that foods are demagnetized when they are cooked, and that only living (raw, uncooked) plant foods have the magnetic properties that are needed by the body. He states that the fiber we consume in our diets should be comprised of the fiber or roughage of raw plant foods, and that if this fiber comes from cooked foods, it will be demagnetized, or devitalized, to the extent that it will pass through the system with little or no benefit.

In addition, cooked, starchy foods leave a plaster-like coating on the walls of the large intestine (colon). This coating builds up over time as more of these foods are consumed, which decreases the capacity to absorb vital nutrients and prevents food from being completely digested. More is provided about this in the next chapter.

Cooked food is any food heated above 118° F. It includes almost every kind of food that comes in an airtight sealed package (bag, box, can, jar, bottle, etc.). For comparison purposes, a hot shower is 105° F, typical pasteurization temperature is 160° F, water boils at 212° F, canned foods are heated during the canning process to 240-250° F, and microwave and stove ovens heat foods to 300-500° F.

"Cooked food is dead, and actually unsuitable as nourishment for the digestive processes of all animals, including human beings." - Dr. Ann Wigmore, <u>Be Your Own Doctor</u>.

Cooked foods (plant or animal) are foods devoid of life. They require additional energy from the body to be digested and assimilated, energy that could be used for other purposes, such as healing. Cooked foods contain coagulated and unusable proteins and dead enzymes that are toxic to the body.

According to Dr. D. C. Jarvis in his book, *Folk Medicine*, cooking reduces potassium 70% for carrots, onions, potatoes, pumpkin and spinach, 60% for cauliflower, cabbage, peas, asparagus, string beans and Brussel sprouts, and 50% for corn, beets and tomatoes. Potassium is needed for the proper functioning of the nervous system.

Cooked foods are tasteless compared to raw foods, which is why they require condiments, such as salt, pepper and sugar, and combinations of them. Many of the condiments have deleterious effects on the body, including sugar and refined salt, as explained in later chapters.

Because cooked foods are dead foods and deficient in nutrients, our hunger is not sated when we eat them in small portions, so we overeat. However, overeating is known to be a precursor of many health complications, including obesity and disease.

As stated previously, raw plant foods are foods as-found in nature. They are not cooked or chemically altered, and they do not contain preservatives, artificial colors or flavors. Raw plant foods are living foods with their natural life force properties intact. It is this life force that is imparted to us when we eat raw plant foods.

The dangers of cooked foods discussed so far are sufficient in themselves to justify eliminating all cooked foods from your diet. But cooking of foods has more dangers. If food is browned by heat treatment, such as by broiling, baking or deep frying, dangerous chemicals are created, such as advanced glycation end-products (AGEs), which have been linked to diabetes and heart disease. This was discussed in a previous chapter.

Furthermore, nutritional experts assert that cooked food is addictive. Like other addictions, the cooked food addiction gets stronger with continued use. Details are provided later in this book on how to kick this addiction.

The consensus of modern nutritional experts, including Norman W. Walker, Robert Morse, Arnold Ehret, Theresa Mitchell, Ann Wigmore, Edward Howell, David Wolfe, Herbert M. Shelton, O.L.M. Abramowski, Fred Hirsch, Harvey Diamond, Bernard Jensen, Professor Spira, Kristina Carrillo-Bucaram, Victoria Boutenko, Joe Alexander and Paavo Airola, is that the consumption of cooked foods is detrimental to human health, and that they should not be eaten.

Enzymes

Enzymes are life-force factors, biological catalysts that are necessary for life processes. They are substances that make life possible. Enzymes are needed for every chemical reaction that takes place in the body. It is claimed that no mineral, vitamin or hormone can do any work without enzymes. The body's ability to digest and assimilate foods is totally dependent on enzymes.

"I attest that the kitchen stove and its big brothers, the heat treatment machinery in food factories, are responsible for destroying a whole category of food elements, namely the heat-sensitive exogenous food enzymes." - Dr. Edward Howell, Enzyme Nutrition.

Raw plant foods are replete with enzymes as provided by nature to facilitate their digestion and assimilation in the body. According to Dr. Edward Howell, raw plant foods have all the enzymes needed for human consumption. The pancreas produces enzymes, but you'll always have exogenous enzymes if you eat raw, uncooked foods.

"To get enzymes from food, one must eat raw food. The heat used in cooking destroys all food enzymes and forces the organism to produce more enzymes, thus enlarging digestive organs, especially the pancreas." - Dr. Edward Howell, Enzyme Nutrition.

The nutritional experts believe that eating cooked food requires the body to use up its enzyme reserves for digestion and assimilation. More specifically, the enzymes of the body must perform the job of digesting cooked foods. This depletes the enzyme reserves of the body, making it increasingly difficult as time goes by to properly digest foods. As a result, we become weaker and more fatigued despite the amount of food we consume. In addition, energy that is used by the body to digest cooked foods is diverted away from other badly needed bodily functions such as self-cleansing and healing.

One of the things that interests me in particular about the dangers of eating cooked foods is that Dr. Howell in his book, Enzyme Nutrition, states that enzyme activity in the body becomes weaker with age. He also states that based on clinical studies performed on animals and humans, each of us is given a limited supply of enzymes at birth, and that when the supply is depleted, we die, and the faster we use up our enzyme supply the shorter our life will be. This is one of the main reasons why we should avoid all cooked foods. It implies that the more cooked foods we eat, the sooner our life will come to an end.

Again, cooked foods are devoid of enzymes because heat destroys them. Furthermore, cooked foods cause us to look older than we really are. They make wrinkles appear, especially on the face.

Dr. Ann Wigmore, in her book, *Be Your Own Doctor*, states that when food is cooked it permits tumors and cancer growth to build, but when food is eaten raw the cancer and other growths immediately begin to shrink. This indicates that cooked foods are precursors of human disease.

As mentioned in the chapter on "What Foods Should We Eat and Why," there is a dearth of information on the Web regarding the dangers of eating cooked foods. Many of the websites queried for this information actually encourage the eating of cooked foods as part of a healthy diet. Again, books have the answers to the really tough nutritional issues.

Raw plant foods may be sliced, diced, run through a food processor, blender, etc., as long as they are not cooked. They can be eaten by themselves or combined with other raw foods if properly combined (see chapter on "Proper Food Combinations").

"Eating raw foods is the number one activity which preserves enzymes and maximizes health." - Gabriel Cousens, <u>Conscious Eating</u>.

The conclusion of this chapter is obvious. We should eat as many enzyme-rich foods as possible, which are raw plant foods, and avoid all cooked foods.

Vegetables that are so often cooked can be eaten raw. We can eat raw potatoes, as long as we don't eat green ones that can be toxic. Also, there are plenty of raw plant foods that satisfy cravings for cooked foods and sweets. For example, what is more satisfying than a ripe peach or mango? You can snack on pecans and honey, cacao nibs or bee pollen soaked in water, bananas with Mission figs or dates and sweet apples.

The dangers of eating cooked foods may shock or surprise many people because most of us grew up eating cooked foods and have learned to like them. Hopefully, this chapter will serve as a re-thinking starting point about how cooked foods should be viewed.

Substituting living plant foods for cooked foods solves all of the problems described in this chapter.

For more information about how cooked foods are harmful to human health, I refer you to the books listed in the Bibliography by Norman W. Walker, Robert Morse, Arnold Ehret, Theresa Mitchell, Ann Wigmore, Edward Howell, David Wolfe, Herbert M. Shelton, O.L.M. Abramowski, Fred Hirsch, Harvey Diamond, Bernard Jensen, Professor Spira, Kristina Carrillo-Bucaram, Victoria Boutenko, Joe Alexander and Paavo Airola.

The Dangers of Starchy Foods

Two of the most eminent nutritionists of recent times, Professor Arnold Ehret and Dr. Norman W. Walker, made remarkable discoveries of how starchy foods harm the body. They discovered that patients who habitually eat starchy foods, including pastries and other bread products,, rice, and pasta have clogged up intestines, and. furthermore, that it was the cause of their diseased conditions.

Any starchy food, including macaroni, pizza and potatoes, can be made into paste or plaster. Many of us know this. But what many of us may not know is that the same foods can cause intestinal obstruction to the point where the passage of the wastes becomes completely cut off.

Through X-rays taken of the large intestines of patients, as well as autopsies, Dr. Norman W. Walker discovered that the obstructions increase in thickness over time and were caused by the starch plating out on the intestinal lining. The plate-out coated lining of the intestines prevents nutrient exchange in the bloodstream. It causes constipation. In time, it builds up to where the passage of waste is greatly reduced, or even cut off completely, requiring hospitalization and surgery -- which often means colostomy.

In other words, constipation caused by starchy foods can be so severe that all waste can be prevented from being expelled from the body. The severe bodily toxicity that such a condition produces causes sickness and disease.

Walker believed that any treatment of disease would be totally ineffective unless the accumulated starchy plaque that has formed in the large intestine over the years has been washed out of the colon by colonic irrigations. This conclusion is based on his healing of chronically ill patients by having them undergo a series of colonics. It was the cleansing action of the colonics that caused the plaque to be released from the walls of the colon, and when that occurred the health of his patients was restored. This is exactly what Arnold Ehret and others have stressed in their books.

For years I ate whatever foods were sold and whatever I wanted in the days of innocence when I didn't know any better. But I know better now because my quest for living constipation-free has led me to good books about what really causes it and what foods to avoid to be constipation- and disease-free. In fact, as discussed in this book, the two go hand in hand, for when you cure constipation you effectively eliminate one of the main causes of disease. I can feel what starchy foods do to me every time I eat them, so I no longer eat them.

The clogging up of the intestines caused by starchy foods causes intestinal bacteria to multiply inordinately, which releases poisons into the blood stream. The state of constipation is the primary cause of illness and disease in the human body also according to Professor Arnold Ehret, Dr. Ann Wigmore, Fred Hirsch, Karyn Calabrese, Professor Spira, and other noted nutritionists.

Many of the contributors to our understanding of the causes of human diseases were famous nutritionists, including Professor Arnold Ehret, who was popular in Germany in the early 1900s, and later in America.

Ehret was probably the first scientist to recognize that mucus-forming foods cause waste obstruction in the body, and that the obstruction causes disease. In his book, *The Cause and Cure of Human Illness,* he states that there are two main reasons for human disease: 1) constipation caused by mucus-producing foods, and 2) overeating, i.e., eating more than is necessary, more than the system can handle, more than it actually needs.

In his landmark book, *The Mucusless Diet Healing System*, first published in 1922, Ehret released to the world his incredible findings about how optimum health can be achieved by eating a starch-free diet consisting of fresh raw fruits, leafy greens and non-starchy vegetables (mucusless foods) which he claimed was the optimal diet for human health. These are the natural foods of man (Genesis' "fruits and herbs"). The book is considered by many nutritional experts to be the definitive work on the prevention and curing of human disease through diet and fasting.

Ehret healed himself of Bright's disease (a kidney disease), and cured many hopeless cases of chronic diseases by putting his patients on his mucusless diet and fasting regimen. Many of the patients were very serious cases with terminal diseases, and lay on their deathbeds. Many had gone through other therapies and followed the advice given, including strict diets, but without success. He also cured those who suffered from degenerative diseases, both acute and chronic. After following his mucusless diet for only a short time, all of his patients regained their health.

As stated in the chapter on "What Foods Should We Eat and Why?", starchy foods include wheat, corn, rice, white and red potatoes, but also beans of all kinds and peas. They also include food products made from these foods, such as bread, pasta, cereals, pastries, corn starch, etc. (Note that carrots and beets are non-starchy foods as discussed in the chapter on "Proper Food Combinations.")

Many people are not aware of the dangers of starchy foods, as they are not aware of the dangers of cooked foods. At the time of this writing, I could not find any websites that discussed the harmful effects that starches have on the large intestine (colon), or that attribute starchy foods to causing disease.

"If you consumed a lifetime supply of dairy, meat and other mucus-producing foods, you may have built up many layers of glue-like toxins on your colon walls. Although some waste can pass through your intestines daily, leading you to believe that your body is adequately digesting the food you eat, the lining of your intestines will continue to toughen and narrow." - Karyn Calabrese, Soak Your Nuts.

"No system of healing can be permanently effective until the eliminative organs have been thoroughly cleansed of accumulated waste matter and at the same time all grain and starchy foods have been eliminated from one's diet." - Norman W. Walker, Become Younger.

The clogging up process resulting from the consumption of starchy foods can be easily proven on a whole plant food diet like the raw vegan diet by simply eating white flour products, such as pizza or while flour bread, for one or more days. The result is constipation and difficult bowel movements, whereas avoiding these foods results in the return of regular and smooth defecations.

Let me ask you a simple question. Are you sure you want to eat that next slice of bread or bowl of rice?

Abiding by Nature's Laws

Natural laws govern our world. They include the laws of physics that encompass the mysterious forces of electromagnetism, gravity and the nuclear forces, and also the laws of biological processes, including life itself. Natural laws are always in effect, and they apply to everyone in every generation.

All creatures seem to be perfectly attuned and adjusted to these laws, except for man. We are constantly challenging or testing Nature in one way or another. Our free will, which other creatures do not have, and which sets us apart from the other creatures perhaps more than anything else, enables us to question the validity of natural laws. But Nature has a way of punishing and even eliminating people who break her laws.

In the province of Nature, things happen to us as a consequence of the way that we choose to live, including our food choices and eating habits. For example, if I combine my foods improperly, I can expect to get a stomachache or headache. If I eat the Standard American Diet, I can expect to be the recipient of a large number of food-related health disorders that are linked to meat and dairy products and to devitalized, refined and processed foods.

The law of cause and effect is one of Nature's laws. It happens to be the foundation of the scientific method, which is the basis for all the discoveries and inventions made in the sciences, including chemistry, physics, geology, biology and the medical sciences. The law of cause and effect is observed in many clinical trials and studies that are conducted on human health and nutrition each year that show a direct relationship between the diseases of humankind and diet. Some of these trials and studies are documented in articles of the scientific and medical professions, many of which are available on the Internet, and some are cited in this book as well as in the books that are listed in the Bibliography.

If you don't want the effect, do something about the causes.

"The present ignorance of the laws underlying normal health is now, in this century, the greatest of all the past centuries, and is evidenced by the deterioration of the so-called civilized people health-wise." - Arnold Ehret, Physical Fitness Through a Superior Diet, Fasting, and Dietetics.

As discussed in previous chapters, many medical researchers and nutritionists claim that the cause of many human diseases are the foods that are commonly consumed, rather than normal processes of aging, such as natural "wear and tear" of the body. It is my belief that this claim will be proven to everyone's satisfaction in the years to come, impacting many popular beliefs regarding age-related health issues. An example is the degenerative disease of arthritis. Many nutritionists, including Dr. Ann Wigmore, believe that arthritis is caused by harmful dietary practices.

Raw plant foods have their enzymes intact to assist the body in their digestion, but cooking destroys food enzymes. The lack of enzymes in cooked foods causes the body to draw on its enzyme reserves for their digestion. Many nutritionists, such as Dr. Edward Howell, contend that this is one of the causes of degeneration in the body.

"Among the many thousands of species of creatures living on the earth, only humans and some of their domesticated animals (dogs, cats) try to live without food enzymes. And only these transgressors of nature's laws are penalized with defective health." - Dr. Edward Howell, Enzyme Nutrition.

Fasting (simply eating less) is one of Nature's powerful ways of cleansing the body of the harmful effects of improper diet and too much eating. When animals get sick, they instinctively abstain from food. But man seems to have lost this instinct, if he ever had it.

It is our duty to understand Nature's laws if we wish to live a healthy life, one that is free of health disorders, including diseases. The appreciation of the power of a natural law at work in us is one of the most profound things that we can ever experience.

Eating foods with their enzymes intact undestroyed by heal (i.e., raw plant foods), avoiding the dangers of cooked and starchy foods, practicing proper food combinations, and curing health issues through a combination of proper diet and fasting are only a few examples of dietary practices that adhere to the laws of Nature. You will learn about these things, and more, in this book.

Another law of nature is the need for adequate rest. In our fast-paced society, with its unrelenting demands on our time and money, our minds cry out for adequate rest. We are told that eight hours of sleep per night are required for health, but many of us get less than five. Is this abiding by Nature's laws?

"Health is the inevitable result of a strict obedience to God's physical and natural laws." - Fred S. Hirsch, Internal Cleanliness.

The body always lets us know how we are treating it. Under-standing and heeding the warning signals the body provides helps us to maintain ourselves in concert with the laws of nature. As mentioned previously, the body can take a lot of abuse before it starts to show the ill effects of deterioration. But when that occurs, a person could be, health-wise speaking, at the point of no return. By staying proactive in this regard, we can avoid many of the health disorders, including diseases, that stalk our society.

This reveals a basic truth about our lives. The longer-term consequences of our choices may be different than their immediate effects. To avoid the perils of constipation, one must not eat foods that cause it, notwithstanding the joy one may have in doing so.

"Healing is no accident. All nature heals itself when causes are removed and the conditions of health supplied." - Dr. Herbert M. Shelton.

Proper Food Combinations

"Cook not, neither mix all things one with another, lest your bowels become as steaming bogs...for I tell you truly, if you mix together all sorts of food in your body, then the peace of your body will cease, and endless war will rage in you." - Attributed to Jesus, The Essene Gospel of Peace, Book One.

Before food can nourish the body, it must be digested. Digestion is a chemical process that breaks down food into constituents that can be assimilated by the body. Digestion starts in the mouth with saliva and continues in the stomach where digestive juices, or gastric juices, are secreted to break down the food. The job of digestion is not finished until the food travels through the small and large intestines and the wastes pass out of the body.

Food combination laws are rules of nature that are based on the principle that different types of foods require different times for digestion, and cause the secretion in the stomach of different types of gastric juices, some being more acidic, some less acidic. If we eat foods that cause more alkaline (less acidic) gastric juices for their digestion together with foods that require more acidic juices for their digestion, the juices combine, resulting in food in the stomach that is difficult to digest. This leads to a variety of complications, such as stomachaches, headaches and fermentation, and, when the food passes through the intestines, putrefaction, gas and the breeding of parasites.

When foods are difficult to digest, the energy reserves of the body are called into play to assist in the job of digestion. It should not be surprising that you feel tired after eating a big meal of improperly combined foods – the traditional nap after a Thanksgiving dinner.

The stomach does not decide what foods to put in it. It leaves that job to the brain.

The Web adequately covers many aspects of proper food combining. A good website on proper food combining at the time of this writing is: https://www.acidalkalinediet.net/correct-food-combining-principles.php.

However, some Web articles on food combining do not stand up to careful scrutiny. For example, some tell us that combining nuts with sweet fruits is an improper food combination. But based on my experience, and what nutritional experts tell us, fatty nuts (like walnuts and pecans) combine well with some sweet fruits, such as bananas and dates. Other sweet fruits, such as apples; that have a high water content, can make the nuts indigestible.

In *The Sunfood Diet Success System*, David Wolfe explains that nuts are actually fat-dominant, not protein-dominant, foods because they consist mostly of fat (see the table provided in the chapter "The Foods We Should Eat and Why"). He explains that the fat in nuts and seeds allows the natural sugar in sweet fruit to be time-released, which helps digestion and provides more long-term energy. Combining sweet fruits with fatty nuts and seeds is an acceptable food combination, contrary to some of the articles on the Web.

The food combination laws should be learned, even if one or two of them are not correctly stated on the Web. The laws that are not correctly stated on the Web at least err on the safe side so that by observing them you will not be hurting yourself. Set goals for yourself to rigidly put the laws into practice.

The rules of food combining are soundly rooted in physiology and thoroughly tested by experience.

"More than sixty years spent in feeding the well and the sick, the weak and the strong, the old and the young, have demonstrated that a change to correctly combined meals is followed by an immediate improvement in health as a consequence of lightening the load the digestive organs have to carry, thus assuring better digestion." - Herbert M. Shelton, <u>Food Combining Made Easy</u>.

I enjoy many foods by themselves, but I'm an inveterate mixer. I prefer to mix my foods, to combine them. I learned the food combination laws the hard way, by trial and error, and suffered all the resulting stomachaches of improperly combined foods. Very probably, you will learn them the hard way too. It took me about a year to put the laws into practice without making further mistakes.

Five of the food combination laws that are important on any diet, including the raw vegan diet, are as follows.

1. Don't Eat Proteins with Starches

Example: Spirulina or hemp seed (both protein foods) eaten with Maca (a starchy food).

2. Don't Eat Starches with Acid Fruit

Example: Potatoes or peas (both starchy foods) eaten with tomatoes (acid fruit).

Note that tomatoes combine well with leafy greens and fatty plant foods like avocados.

3. Don't Eat Starches with Sweet or Sub-Acid Fruit

Example: Beans or peas (starchy foods) added to green smoothies that contain sweet or sub-acid fruit.

I have my own rule for this – don't add vegetables other than leafy greens to green smoothies. I've had too many stomachaches from breaking this law, so I make it easier to remember by excluding all vegetables (except greens) from my green smoothies which contain sweet fruit.

4. Don't Eat Sweet Fruit with Acid Fruit

Example: Pineapple (an acid fruit) eaten with bananas or dates (sweet fruit).

Note that sweet fruit combines well with sub-acid fruits, e.g., apricots.

5. Don't Eat Proteins with Sweet Fruit

Example: Hemp seed with dates. Hemp seed is 30% protein. Higher protein foods, such as spirulina, are even worse combinations with sweet fruit because they cause severe gas resulting from the fermentation that occurs. Bananas are an exception because they combine well with nuts and seeds.

The above food combination laws cover some of the errors typically made on the raw vegan diet. Additional food combination laws should also be learned. As explained previously, you can learn about them on the Web.

Greens (green leafy vegetables) are the only foods that combine well with all other foods, including other greens.

To aid in preparing meals, the digestion times required for different types of foods should also be learned. Obviously, we should not combine foods that require completely different digestion times. Digestion times for different foods are adequately covered on the Web. Typically, digestion times and proper food combinations go hand in hand.

When the food combination laws are obeyed, digestion is greatly improved and overall well-being is enhanced. When food combination laws are broken, stomachaches, headaches, excessive flatulence, or other complications can and do result, which can quickly turn what started out to be a good day into a bad one.

"Improved digestion results in general improvement in all the functions of life. Many and great are the benefits to flow from improved digestion." - Dr. Herbert M. Shelton, <u>Food Combining Made Easy</u>.

How to Determine the Starch Content of Foods

Food labels (Nutrition Facts Labels) typically give the amount of total carbohydrates, sugar and fiber but not the amount of starch in the food. The starch content might be published on the Web, but if it's not, here's how to determine the starch content of any food from its Nutrition Facts Label.

From the food label on the product package, or as given on the Web, get the weights in grams of total carbohydrates, sugars and fiber and plug them into the following equation:

Starch = Carbs – (Sugars + Fiber).

Example 1: Maca. On the Web, the Nutrition Facts Label for Maca lists, for a 100g serving: 71g carbs, 32g sugars and 7g fiber.

Starch (g) = 71g – (32g + 7g) = 71g – 39g = 32g

32g/100g = 32%

Maca is 32% starch. Since starch content is a considerable portion of Maca, it is a starchy vegetable.

Example 2: Carrots. Per the Web, a 61g serving of carrots has 6g carbs, 2.9g sugars and 1.7g fiber.

Starch (g) = 6g – (2.9g + 1.7g) = 6g – 4.8g = 1.2g

1.2g/61g = 2%

Carrots are 2% starch. Since the starch content of carrots is very low, it is a non-starchy vegetable.

Many articles on the Web differ on whether carrots are starchy or non-starchy vegetables. Some articles say carrots are starchy vegetables while others say they are non-starchy vegetables. This is another example of conflicting information found on the Web.

Example 3: **Beets**. Per the Web, a 100g serving of beets has 10g carbs, 7g sugars and 2.8g fiber.

Similar to the above computations, beets are 0.2% starch. It is a non-starchy vegetable.

Example 4: **Turnips**. Per the Web, a 122g serving of turnips has 8g carbs, 4.6g sugars and 2.2g fiber.

Similar to the above computations, turnips are 0.1% starch. It is a non-starchy vegetable.

Example 5: **Cinnamon**. Per the Web, a 7.8g serving of cinnamon has: 6g carbs, 4.1g sugars and 0.2g fiber.

Similar to the above computations, cinnamon is 21% starch. Cinnamon is a starchy food. It should not be used with protein foods or with sweet or sub-acid fruit.

As the proper combination of hydrocarbons in your vehicle's fuel determines how it runs, so your life will run smoothly if your foods are eaten in their proper combinations. In my opinion, if positive feedback is not received by the body on any food that is eaten, no matter what the type or variety – fruit, vegetable, Superfood, herb or any other kind of food – then that food should either be eaten in a more ripe condition, in smaller quantities, in proper combinations with other foods, or it should be avoided. The body is no fool. It recognizes foods that disagree with it or do it harm by giving us warning signals. Our job then is to correctly interpret these signals.

Longevity

Alchemists, scientists and laymen throughout history have tried to discover the secrets of longevity, or a long life. It was once believed that all one had to do was to find the "Elixir of Life," which was thought to be a certain food or mixture of foods that would bestow eternal youth on its possessor.

The Holy Scriptures appear to be the origin of the belief that there once was an Elixir of Life. In Genesis 1:29, God gave to mankind a diet consisting of whole plant foods, which is best described as the raw vegan diet. But there were two trees in the Garden of Eden that had special fruit; one was the tree of good and evil, and the other was the tree of life, a tree that would make man live forever.

Genesis 2:9:
"And out of the ground the Lord God made every tree grow that is pleasant to the sight and good for food. The tree of life was also in the midst of the garden, and the tree of the knowledge of good and evil."

Genesis 3:22:
"Then the Lord God said, "Behold, the man has become like one of Us, to know good and evil. And now, lest he put out his hand and take also of the tree of life, and eat, and live forever –."

Genesis 3:24:
"So He drove out the man; and He placed cherubim at the east of the garden of Eden, and a flaming sword which turned every way, to guard the way to the tree of life."

Many seekers of long life have wondered what kind of food grew on the Tree of Life. As far as we know, no one has succeeded in identifying it or what is probably the same thing, the Elixir of Life. But sometimes beliefs are hard to dispel, especially when they are based on truth.

Everyone wants to live longer, whether for putting things to right or for enjoyment. However, not everyone knows how to go about ensuring their longevity.

One of the great contributors to our understanding of how to live a long life was Luigi Cornaro, a nobleman who lived in Italy during the fifteenth and sixteenth centuries. His remarkable books include *Sure Methods of Attaining a long and Healthful Life*, *The Surest Method of Correcting an Infirm Constitution*, and *How to Live 100 Years, or Discourses on the Sober Life*. His books are listed in the Bibliography.

The term that Cornaro used in his books to describe how to attain long life through optimum health was "sobriety." By sobriety he meant the following:

"Sobriety is reduced to two things, quality and quantity. The first consists in avoiding food or drinks which are found to disagree with the stomach. The second, to avoid taking more than the stomach can easily digest." - Luigi Cornaro, <u>How to Live 100 Years, or Discourses on the Sober Life</u>.

According to his books, Cornaro ate very sparingly each and every day of his life, after curing himself in his 40s of maladies that his doctors said would soon cause his death. In his later years he never overate but always under-ate.

As discussed in the chapter on "What Foods Should We Eat and Why?", immediately after the Flood, when animal food was permitted to be eaten, the average human lifespan fell from about 900 years to about 400 years. Today, according to the latest worldwide statistics, the average human lifespan is 72 years. What does this indicate? It indicates a slow decline in human longevity based on a departure from the God-given diet.

Luigi Cornaro lived to 102. What does it tell us about the importance of reducing the quantity of food that we eat, as well as fasting between meals which he obviously did by eating so sparingly? According to his books, Cornaro never needed spectacles (glasses), his hearing remained unimpaired, and he could climb hills effortlessly until he died. And he kept his mind sharp by learning new things.

In the last two hundred years, many investigators have studied extended human lifespans by visiting various cultures of the world. They have tried to ascertain why certain peoples lived longer than others. They have performed clinical studies and determined that the centenarians (those who were at least 100 years old) had the following things in common.

- They were moderate or light eaters
- They ate very little butter or salt
- They ate little, if any, meat
- They ate fresh foods
- They kept up strenuous activity throughout their lives
- They liked to do outside work and rose early

"The major characteristic of the diet of longevous people is low total calorie intake throughout life." - Dan Georgakas, The Methuselah Factors.

Some of the clinical studies we have of extended human lifespan are documented in the books that are listed in the Bibliography, including *The Methuselah Factors* by Dan Georgakas, *Youth in Old Age* by Alexander Leaf, and *Healthy Aging* by Andrew Weil.

It was only during the last century that nutritionists concluded that the closer an organism (animal or human) comes to its minimal daily food requirements, the longer its lifespan will be. ."

Dr. N.W. Walker, whose books are listed in the Bibliography, spent most of his life exploring man's capability to extend life. He lived to be 99 according to the Web, but some sources say 109. His books are referred to several times in this book since they provide much insight into what foods should be eaten for longevity and optimum health.

According to Dr. Walker, the foods that people should eat for longevity are the foods of the raw vegan diet. Raw plant foods are the most conducive of any foods to longevity because they contain an abundance of life force properties and enzymes and do not contain man-made or -altered ingredients.

Maybe we are only now beginning to understand how to achieve longevity. As discussed in the chapter on "The Dangers of Cooked Foods," enzymes are important life catalysts that are abundant in raw plant foods. Dr. Ann Wigmore, whose books are listed in the Bibliography, believed that enzyme preservation is the secret to longevity.

"Enzymes, apparently, are the key to longevity; they seem to neutralize the basic causes of aging and enable the body to retain its youthful qualities." - Dr. Ann Wigmore, Be Your Own Doctor.

It is our duty to strive for optimum health while we remain in the world of the living. No one knows the day of their death. Happily, we have nothing to do with that date; only God knows its appointed time. But we must be good stewards of our lives and do what is right to promote and sustain our health.

If you seek to extend the term of your existence, then adopt the raw vegan diet, keep physically and mentally active and do not overeat.

Distilled Water

"Pure distilled water is truly God's greatest gift to us, a source of life and health." - Paul C. Bragg.

Drinking distilled water has received a bad rap over the years. This chapter explains why distilled water is, in fact, beneficial to human health and should be the water of choice for all who strive for optimum health.

Contrary to popular belief/misconception, our blood is not comprised of regular water. Human blood is comprised of about 78% fluid, and 90% of it is distilled water. According to nutritional experts, including Dr. N. W. Walker, Paul C. Bragg, and Dr. Allen E. Banik (who spent most of his life researching the effects of water on the human body), we do not need regular water to sustain health, and, more significantly, regular water is harmful to human health. This startling contention is explored in this chapter.

As we progress in our understanding of foods and nutrition, many of the things that humankind has taken for granted throughout the centuries may be exposed as untruths or falsehoods.

Regular water, which includes tap or faucet water, drinking-fountain water, spring, well, river and lake water, is water that has been in contact with the rocks and soil. It also includes filtered water since minerals in regular water are in solution and do not get filtered out. What we normally refer to as "water" includes all of the aforementioned types. They contain inorganic minerals, such as lime (calcium), sodium, iron, phosphorus, magnesium, etc., that have been collected from the rocks or soil that the water has been in contact with.

Distilled water has no inorganic minerals and is devoid of chlorination and fluoridation, heavy metals and pesticides. It is the type of water most compatible with the human body's cells. It is entirely safe for human consumption, and ideally meets the needs of the body.

Also, contrary to popular belief/misconception, distilled water does not leach out minerals that have become part of the body's cells. This in confirmed in Robert Morse's book, *The Detox Miracle Sourcebook*, which states that distilled water dissolves inorganic minerals that are lodged in the tissues and joints of the body, and greatly assists in removing them from the body, but it does not cause minerals that are part of the body's cells to be leached out. Dr. N. W. Walker in his book, *Water Can Undermine Your Health*, states the following:

"It is virtually impossible for distilled water to separate minerals which have become an integral part of the cells and tissues of the body. Distilled water collects only the minerals which remain in the body, minerals discarded from natural water and from the cells, the minerals which the natural water originally collected from its contact with the earth and the rocks. Such minerals, having been rejected by the cells of the body are of no constructive value. On the contrary, they are debris which distilled water is capable of picking up and eliminating from the system." – Dr. N. W. Walker, Water Can Undermine Your Health.

Again, distilled water cannot leach out minerals that have become part of the body's cells. What it can do is leach out excess minerals that are deposited in the joints and tissues of the body, minerals that the body could not properly utilize.

"Distilled water acts as a solvent in the body. It dissolves food substances so they can be assimilated and taken into every cell. It dissolves inorganic mineral substances lodged in tissues of the body so that such substances can be eliminated in the process of purifying the body. Distilled water is the greatest solvent on earth, the only one that can be taken into the body without damage to the tissues. By its continued use, it is possible to dissolve inorganic minerals, acid crystals, and all the other waste products of the body without injuring tissues." - Dr. Allen E. Banik, The Choice is Clear.

Organic minerals are the minerals we get from eating plants. Plants convert the inorganic minerals found in the water that they take up from the soil into a readily usable-by-the-body organic form. Organic minerals are not deposited in the tissues and joints of the body but are utilized by the cells of the body for their regeneration.

Distilled water is regular, hard water that has been condensed after the water is boiled. Distillation is the most effective method of purifying water. The minerals stay behind because they are not volatile, and the condensed steam is pure of minerals, bacteria, viruses and physical impurities. Even rain water is not as pure as distilled water since it contains impurities picked up by the rain from the air.

Since the time that municipal water was first chlorinated, it has been maintained by many that drinking regular water, the water that originates from streams and lakes, which includes municipal recycled water, mineral waters and bottled waters, is good for health because it has minerals the body needs. However, according to many nutritionists, inorganic minerals that are contained in regular water should not be put into the human body.

"There is only one way you can purify your body and help to eliminate your chronic aging diseases and that is through the miracle of distilled water." - Dr. Allen E. Banik, <u>The Choice is Clear.</u>

In addition to lacking inorganic minerals, distilled water is totally lacking in dangerous metals and chemicals that are found in today's drinking and bottled waters.

Paul and Patricia Bragg, in their book *Water, The Shocking Truth That Can Change Your Life*, state that the tap water we use for cooking, bathing and drinking can be responsible for many ailments because of the addition of harmful chemicals such as sodium fluoride and chlorine. The book explains the dangers of these chemicals. The authors further state that distilled water is the only water we should drink, not only because it removes inorganic mineral deposits and toxins from the joints of the body, but because it helps remove cholesterol and fat.

"Inorganic minerals, toxic chemicals, fluoride and contaminants can pollute, clog up and even turn tissues to stone throughout your body, causing pain, illness and even premature death!" - Paul C. Bragg, <u>Water, The Shocking Truth That Can Save Your Life</u>.

For similar reasons, Dr. N. W. Walker, in his many books, states that distilled water should be used for cooking and drinking.

"Distilled water is always the safest to drink. As regular water may leave deposits of calcium and other unwanted minerals in the blood circulation, these may find their way into the endocrine gland system with disastrous results which might never be attributed to these unusable minerals as the cause." - Norman W. Walker, <u>Water Can Undermine Your Health</u>.

Some people have purchased reverse osmosis water filtration units for under-the-sink home use to purify their faucet water for drinking or cooking purposes. In the reverse osmosis process, water is purified by forcing a portion of the faucet water through a semi-permeable membrane. The process removes a high percentage of the dissolved solids as well as other contaminants from the water. However, Dr. Allen E. Banik, in his book, *The Choice is Clear*, explains why reverse osmosis water is not preferable to distilled water, in the following excerpt:

"While the result [of reverse osmosis] often approaches the purity of distilled water. the degree of purity in any case varies widely, depending on the types and conditions of the equipment used, much as with filter equipment, and the effectiveness lessens with use, sometimes drastically!" - Dr. Allen E. Banik, <u>The Choice is Clear</u>.

The advantages of drinking distilled water are many as described above. From my researching, I did not find any disadvantages except for what appears on websites. For the websites that were polled for this information, I did not find any that supported the claims of the nutritionists that have been cited in this chapter. Once again, this exemplifies the disconnect that exists between the truths about foods and nutrition versus the claims on popular media.

I have been drinking distilled water for years with absolutely no ill effects. I switched from hard, faucet and bottle waters to distilled water when I read the books that describe the health benefits of drinking distilled water. I find its taste to be much better than faucet water or bottled waters, and I can testify to the positive difference it makes in my health.

My recommendation is that everyone on the raw vegan diet switch to drinking distilled water for their health. The next time you are shopping for bottled water, pick up a gallon of distilled water instead. At the time of this writing, distilled water was selling for about eighty cents per gallon at retail stores like Wal-Mart.

Within the first month of drinking distilled water, I noticed a marked increase in my thirst for the water. Previously, it seemed that I never drank very much water and I never liked the taste of it when I drank it. But now, I love the taste of water in its purist form, with its thirst-quenching ability as a bonus. Distilled water is, for me, a truly rewarding experience. There is something about distilled water and the actions it performs on the body that are very remarkable. Distilled water is what I believe the body craves.

It is said that the older we get the more we lose our ability to sense thirst. As a result, our bodies become more and more dehydrated as we continue to age, without us being able to recognize it. This chronic dehydration can cause serious health problems.

"Chronic and persistently increasing dehydration is the root cause of almost all currently encountered diseases of the human body." - F. Batmanghelidj, M.D, Your Body's Many Cries for Water.

What has changed my life more than anything else in recent years has been switching to the raw vegan diet and drinking distilled water.

The Good and Bad About Salt

Salt (sodium chloride) is essential to life. The Romans paid their troops in salt, hence the word "salary." Our bodies need salt, but there are different kinds of salt and some have proven to be harmful to the body.

Robert O. Young and Shelley R. Young, in their book, *The pH Miracle*, describe the differences between what they consider to be "bad salt" and "good salt." "Bad salt" is common table salt, the salt that is widely used in homes and restaurants in America and throughout the world, and is the salt commonly added to refined and processed foods. Let's talk about table salt before discussing the "good salt."

Nutritional experts and even members of the medical profession have implicated table salt with the high incidence of high blood pressure and kidney problems in the Western world. Table salt is unnatural, highly-refined salt that has been heat treated to very high temperatures which alters the chemical structure of the salt. The salt is then bleached white and combined with anti-caking agents, fluoride, dextrose, aluminum hydroxide (to improve its pour-ability) and preservatives. Aluminum is widely recognized as a neurotoxin and a potential cause of Alzheimer's disease. An easy way to recognize refined salt is its bleached white color.

As explained in *The pH Miracle,* many of the additives in table salt, such as those listed above, are not required to be listed on food labels, including the food labels on canned, bottled and jarred (refined and processed) foods and the food labels on packages of salt. These labels typically just list "salt" as an ingredient.

The Web has some good articles about the health hazards of table salt. For example, search on "common table salt health" or "table salt poison."

F. Batmanghelidj, M.D, in his book, *Your Body's Many Cries for Salt,* states that the salt we use should be unrefined sea salt.

Jacques de Langre in his book, *Sea Salt's Hidden Powers*, states that refined and processed salt has an altered chemical structure and lacks the electrolytic positive and negative charge properties that natural sea salt possesses.

Many products with "sea salt" as an ingredient actually contain refined sea salt, not unrefined, natural sea salt. I wish I had known that years ago when I used "iodized sea salt" on my foods. *The pH Miracle* states that 89% of all sea salt commercially sold has been refined and processed, that is, its chemical structure has been altered by extreme heat and chemicals have been added. Like table salt, refined sea salt is always bleached white in color. The sea salt I was using for years was bright white in color.

Natural sea salt, the kind that comes from evaporating sea water by the heat of the sun, is not refined, meaning that it has not been heat treated by modern refining techniques, and it does not contain man-made additives. It is not blanched white like refined salts, but has a natural grayish or pinkish cast to it.

There are several commercially available natural sea salts to choose from. An example is Celtic Sea Salt, which is a North Atlantic Ocean sun-evaporated salt. It contains over 80 minerals and is considered a full-spectrum natural sea salt. Other brands include Pink Himalayan Sea Salt and Real Salt, both of which are mined from salt deposits in the earth that apparently were formed by the Biblical Flood. Pink Himalayan sea salt comes from Pakistan. and Real Salt comes from Utah. You can learn more about these salts on the Web.

F. Batmanghelidj in his book (referenced above) states that there are hidden "miracles" in unrefined sea salt. These include:

• Extracting excess acidity from the cells of the body, particularly the brain cells.

• Preserving the serotonin and melatonin levels in the brain.

• It is vital for the communication and information processing of nerve cells.

• Salt and water perform natural antioxidant duties and clear toxic waste from the body.

• Maintaining muscle tone and strength, reduces stress and emotional disorders and assists sleep.

"A salt-free diet is utterly stupid." - F. Batmanghelidj, <u>Your Body's Many Cries for Salt</u>.

One of the leading experts on foods and nutrition in the world today is undoubtedly David Wolfe. Some of his books are listed in the Bibliography. There is probably no one who has eaten as many different kinds of raw plant foods, or has used as many different kinds of natural sea salt, as he. For additional information about sea salt, see David Wolfe's YouTube videos on salt.

Arnold Ehret, in his book, *The Mucusless Diet Healing System*, states that salt is a very good mucus dissolver.

Despite all the good that is reported about using natural sea salt, the fact remains that sea salt is an inorganic salt. Most nutritionists assert that the body cannot effectively utilize inorganic minerals of any kind (e.g., iodine, sodium, calcium, iron, phosphorus, magnesium, etc.). They also assert that inorganic minerals not eliminated by normal bodily processes get stored in the body's tissues and joints. Nutritionists, including those referenced in this book, firmly believe that we should get all our minerals from plants.

"Inorganic minerals are not completely purged from the body by the kidneys and other body organs – only a portion of them are. The rest accumulate in the body tissues and joints. Over time, this accumulation of inorganic minerals results in various degenerative diseases, including arthritis. This accumulation is also said to be the cause of a general enfeebled rigidity called "old age." - N. W. Walker, <u>Water Can Undermine Your Health</u>.

As discussed previously, plants transform inorganic minerals from the soil and also the ocean into organic form that is easily assimilated by the body. Organic salt is contained in vegetables, including sea vegetables, and is what the body needs for health.

"The bottom line is this – no matter where or how on earth it comes from, if salt is not first transformed by plants from inorganic sodium into organic sodium, it can't be properly absorbed by the body!" - Paul C. Bragg, <u>Water, The Shocking Truth That Can Save Your Life</u>.

On a whole plant food diet. there is no lack of mineral salts for electrolyte health. If additional salt is desired because of worries about not getting enough salt, then you should use natural, unrefined sea salt.

Dr. Ann Wigmore in her book, *Be Your Own Doctor*, states that inorganic salts can get deposited in the joints of the body and cause arthritis. She healed herself of arthritis by eliminating table salt from her diet and going on a whole plant food diet.

As explained in N.W Walker's book, *The Natural Way to Vibrant Health*, sea water has all the mineral elements in colloidal (liquid) form. He tells us how he used sea water on his foods with no adverse reactions. It appears that if water is added to natural sea salt and the salt is allowed to dissolve, it would return its minerals to colloidal form as they exist in sea water.

The body needs electrolytes for health. I have been using natural sea salt, such as Celtic Sea Salt and Real Salt, on my vegetables for years without seeing any ill effects. I believe it is due to it being readily assimilated by the body.

The National Academy of Medicine (NAM) recommends limiting salt intake to 1500 mg per day, or about half a teaspoon per day.

I hope that this chapter has provided useful information regarding this important and controversial topic. If you decide to use salt, you should use natural, unrefined sea salt, and use it sparingly.

Proper Eating Habits

"We are not what we eat but what we assimilate" - Paavo O. Airola.

Those who wolf, gulp or bolt down their foods are prone to digestive discomforts and disorders, including heartburn and stomachache to mention only two. Many regularly resort to quick remedies, such as antacids, aspirin and similar drugs. According to the Web, at least $2 billion are spent yearly in the US alone on antacids, and $10 billion worldwide. That's a lot of indigestion!

In addition, many people eat compulsively, often consuming food throughout the day whenever they feel like it whether they're hungry or not. Compulsive eating can be out of habit or because of job-prescribed or tradition-prescribed meal times. If we eat food when we are not hungry, the body is not ready for the food.

These habits are damaging to the human system, and the damage gets worse the more they are practiced. They cannot produce vibrant health because the foods cannot be properly digested and assimilated by the body. Not only do they cause digestive difficulties, but they cause sluggishness and grogginess, general fatigue and various illnesses.

One quarter of what you eat keeps you alive. The other quarter keeps your doctor alive.

Proper eating habits are prescribed by Nature. Food must be eaten in such a way that the full powers of the digestive system are employed. In addition, every ounce of food that passes through the body that is not actually needed by the body is a tax on the body's vital powers, a waste of vital energy.

To avoid these complications and more, most of us need to modify our eating habits.

Digestion occurs primarily in two ways, mechanical digestion and chemical digestion.

Mechanical digestion occurs as the teeth grind and masticate foods. Chewing breaks down food into smaller particles which allow them to be better digested. An old saying is: "Chew your food, your stomach has no teeth."

Chemical digestion begins in the mouth through saliva. The process of chewing activates the flow of saliva. If the mouth does not water during a meal then the digestion of that food is hindered. Some nutritionists claim that food well-salivated is practically half digested before it gets to the stomach. Many raw foodists recommend chewing food until it is liquified in the mouth. When whole plant foods are eaten, the enzymes assist in the chemical digestive process.

Two thousand years ago, Asclepiades of Greece understood that particles of food are a main cause of indigestion. If the particles were small, digestion would follow its normal course, but if the particles were too big, indigestion would occur.

"The chief function of today's cook is to prepare soft pap for the adult, so that little or no chewing is required. Meats are pounded or ground and vegetables cooked to make them easy to swallow with a minimum of chewing; breads are made to be swallowed with very little preliminary mastication; potatoes are mashed, cereals soaked and fruits stewed, so that the muscles of the jaw get very little exercise and the food gets very little saliva. There is no real pleasure in such eating." - Dr. Herbert M. Shelton, Health for the Millions.

To produce the kind of health we want and need to have, the following eating habits should be practiced at every meal.

1. All foods should be eaten slowly, and chewed thoroughly. If you are very hungry before eating, you should still slow down on the eating or the foods will be wolfed or bolted down with little chewing taking place.

2. Do not overeat. This is the cardinal rule to master if you want to obtain optimum health. The best advice I can offer is the same

as that of many others, which is to leave the table when you are 2/3 full. This has often been difficult for me to learn, but I found that when I practiced it everything changed for the better on my journey to optimum health. What it amounts to is, eating only as much as your system actually needs. Only you can determine that. It may take a while to learn, but it is all part of the journey.

"Every individual should, as a general rule, restrain himself to the smallest quantity which he finds from careful investigation, enlightened experience and observation will fully meet the alimentary wants of his system, knowing that whatsoever is more than this is evil." - Dr. Sylvester Graham.

3. Adhere to the proper food combination laws (see the chapter on "Proper Food Combinations.")

4. Make sure fruits are ripe before eating them. How to tell when fruits are ready to be eaten was discussed previously.

5. Enjoy your food! If food is not enjoyed it cannot be efficiently digested. It is why I recommended using a raw vegan dipping sauce for raw vegetables, at least until the food can be enjoyed au naturel, without sauce.

6. If emotionally strung out or upset about something before eating, then skip the meal. Studies have shown that fear, anxiety, tension and anger constrict the entire digestive system and dry up the digestive juices.

7. Limit water or other fluid intake during a meal. It only dilutes the digestive juices that are needed for proper digestion. Drink any liquids at least 1/2 hour before, and no sooner than 1 hour after a meal. Protein and fat meals require the longest times to pass through the stomach (up to 4 hours), so adjust the consumption of liquids after the meal accordingly.

8. Eat to live, instead of live to eat. This was the dictum of Socrates, the most exemplary of the Greek philosophers. It

represents the tried and tested way of health attained by the Greeks during the Golden Age of Athens.

"The rest of the world lives to eat, but I eat to live." - Socrates (470-399 B.C.).

Doing these things, or even only five of them, greatly assists in obtaining the health and vigor we are all seeking.

Transitioning to the Raw Vegan Diet

Professor Arnold Ehret and Dr. N. W. Walker, among others, treated critically and hopelessly ill patients by starting them directly on a raw plant food diet, with no intervening transition period, to save their lives and cure their diseases. Complete cures were achieved under the diet. For more details, see the books by these authors that are listed in the Bibliography.

If you or someone you know is currently facing a serious health crisis such as imminent hospitalization or death, then transitioning to the raw vegan diet may not be appropriate. Instead, I would recommend promptly seeking the advice of a qualified homeopathic or naturopathic professional who is familiar with the healing powers of living plant foods, and getting their opinion on starting directly on the raw vegan diet.

Barring such cases, however, I recommend a gradual, but rather swift transition to the raw vegan diet from whatever diet you may be on. The transition is fully explained in this chapter.

This chapter is intended for all who have not attained the diet that consists of eating uncooked whole plant foods exclusively (i.e., the raw vegan diet), and includes those who are currently on the vegetarian and vegan diets. The difference between these diets is explained below.

Raw plant foods promote optimum health and longevity. They give you the zest and energy you always wanted but never could quite obtain. They make you feel good about each and every day of your life. The raw vegan diet literally transforms you into a new person. Other diets cannot do this.

I recommend transitioning to the raw vegan diet by following, in rapid succession, the order of diets listed below. Transition by first becoming a vegetarian, then a vegan and then a raw vegan. The reasons for this are explained in this chapter.

Vegetarian Diet – The vegetarian diet is a diet that consists mostly of plant foods. It minimizes meat and dairy products but can include some fish, and/or some dairy and poultry such as cheese and eggs. The emphasis of the vegetarian diet is on eating mainly plant foods but also cutting back on animal-based foods. Both cooked plant and animal-based foods are allowed on the vegetarian diet.

Vegan Diet – The vegan diet is somewhat like the vegetarian diet but it goes further to exclude *all* animal-based foods, even fish, cheese and eggs. The vegan diet allows cooked plant foods to be eaten.

Raw Vegan Diet – The raw vegan diet is somewhat like the vegan diet in that it excludes all animal-based foods. But it also excludes all cooked foods, which includes cooked plant foods.

The objective is to attain the raw vegan diet from whatever diet you may currently be on in less than a year. This goal can be achieved even if you are currently on the typical American diet. But it means not wasting anymore time just thinking about switching diets. It means taking the steps necessary to make it happen.

The purpose of the transition period is to learn all that is needed to obtain and maintain the raw vegan diet while suffering the least along the way. Like most changes in life, going through the gears smoothly versus abruptly is easier on the mind and body. You will definitely learn from each of the intermediary diets, but the goal is the raw vegan diet.

It must be emphasized, however, not to dwell in either of the two inferior diets (vegetarian and vegan) for very long. To reach the goal you must keep moving. Plan ahead to go through the two intermediary diets as quickly as possible. The actual time it takes for you to do it will depend on your initiative, persistence and ability to learn new things, but you must keep moving to make it all happen within a year.

You cannot achieve optimal health by making half-hearted attempts at being healthier. This includes remaining on any partially-raw vegan diet like the vegan 80/20 diet (80% raw, 20% cooked) which I was on for a long time. It's like being partially well, which means partially unwell. Actually, the vegan 80/20 diet amounts to being less than 80% well since cooked foods cause toxic buildup in the body tissues which further complicates health. There is no substitute for being 100% healthy. Eating 100% raw plant foods makes you 100% well. Anything short of that does not.

For anyone who is firmly set on eating only raw plant foods starting today, it is possible to jump immediately into the raw vegan diet without a transition period. People have done it. It means quitting harmful foods all at once, which for most people is too big of a change to easily manage, and there are reasons for that.

One of the major obstacles in the way to successfully attaining a whole plant food diet is what I call the curse of "food convenience." Our society is built on fast foods and drinks. We need to break away from these things. It requires shifting our focus to healthy foods and drinks, those with health-appeal rather than taste-appeal. It means taking the time required to shop at local food stores for our foods, even though doing so typically takes only minutes more than it does to drive through a fast food place. This may be a major shift in thinking for many people. It's hard to break old habits. However, they were formed by repetition and they can be broken by repeatedly refraining from them.

The foods we are accustomed to eat have strong ties on us. While we may not always be aware of these ties or attractions, they cause cravings. The transition approach helps to deal with these cravings. But whoever has the resolve and willpower to become a raw vegan without transitioning should definitely go for it. If successful, you will be enjoying the rewards of the raw vegan diet that much sooner.

The knowledge acquired about raw plant foods during this period will make you a smarter shopper and assist you in making better food choices, choices based more on health-appeal than taste-appeal.

An important concept to include in one's thinking about foods is that they are a source of medicine as well as nourishment. When this concept is internalized, great strides in health are possible.

"Let food be thy medicine and medicine be thy food." - Hippocrates.

THINGS TO LEARN DURING THE TRANSITION PERIOD

• The difference between ripe and un-ripe produce.

• Shelf and refrigerator life of most fruits and vegetables.

• What fruits and vegetables can be frozen and not frozen.

• How to read food labels, and what ingredients to avoid.

• The dangers of pesticides.

• The benefits of organic foods.

• The food combination laws.

• What detoxification is, and how to speed up the process.

• How to perform colonics and enemas.

You will learn many of these things by reading this book.

The ancient Roman caution, "Caveat Emptor" ("Let the Buyer Beware"), carries the same weight and significance now as it did in the days of the Roman Empire. It is our responsibility to avoid foods and ingredients that are harmful to us. During the transition period, you will learn to analyze the food labels and understand what they mean.

No matter where you are on the raw vegan diet journey, you can improve your health today simply by quitting one or two harmful foods or ingredients and replacing them with healthier choices. Then, after several weeks, declare victory and move on to quit another food or ingredient, replacing it with a healthier choice. In this way, you progress to the raw vegan diet.

Eliminating all meat and dairy products, refined sugar and refined salt from your diet is a huge step in the right direction. It will be your first goal if you are not already there. It means stop eating fast foods, including energy drinks, sodas and colas, most restaurant foods and refined and processed foods. In the place of meat and dairy products, eat raw fruits, vegetables and leafy greens, and get used to them. Then expand your food selections to include different varieties than those you are already used to. Start using natural, unrefined sea salt (see the chapter on "The Good and Bad About Salt.")

During the transition period, some cooked foods may be eaten. The reason for this is explained below. Remember, however, that the goal is to quit eating cooked foods. Also, my recommendation is to stop eating all starchy foods. Previous chapters of this book have described the dangers of consuming these foods.

Get to where you are eating at least one meal a day of only raw fruit and maybe also greens (e.g., a green smoothie for breakfast). Raw fruits counteract many of the harmful effects of a mixed diet, that is, a cooked food and raw food diet. Eating more raw fruit (fresh or sun-dried) during the transition period will be of benefit to the cells of the body and will enhance the self-cleansing process.

It is during the transition period that the food combination laws are learned. Plan on making mistakes; it's part of any learning experience.

THINGS NEEDED FOR THE RAW VEGAN DIET

- Cutting boards of different sizes

- Knives

- Knife sharpening stone

- Blender

- Lemon/lime squeezer

- Glass or plastic jars with tops (for green smoothies on the go)

If you have never sharpened a knife on a stone, then it's time to learn. A dull knife in the kitchen makes many things more difficult.

I use a reconditioned Vitamix blender and have never had a problem with it. It's probably the only blender I will ever need. Before the Vitamix, I went through several retail store blenders, burning out the motors. Vitamix claims you really have to push the blender to warm foods above 115 degrees F, and I have yet to use it on its maximum speed. The Vitamix container is BPA-free plastic, versus glass, which makes it light weight and easy to clean.

The best lemon/lime squeezer, in my opinion, is a stainless steel, hand-held model. It takes very little pressure to squeeze out the juice of a lemon or lime or other citrus fruit.

Detoxification

Detoxification is the process by which the body auto-cleanses itself of toxic wastes. The body is always trying to purge itself of toxins, but certain foods hinder the process. Detoxification really takes off when raw plant foods are consumed exclusively. If you are on an ordinary diet, the detoxification process is, for all practical purposes, ineffectual because ordinary diets cause toxic wastes to build up to the extent where thorough detoxification is not possible. The detoxification process is also known as self-purification or self-cleansing.

Detoxification is the healthy ridding of the body of its accumulated toxins. The process typically causes more frequent defecations and urinations, and maybe some diarrhea. These things are normal and last only during the cleansing process.

Detoxification is how the body heals and rejuvenates itself. Whole plant foods give the body what it needs for self-cleansing and provide it with the best raw materials for cellular reconstruction. Detoxification is the rite of passage everyone must go through to become genuinely healthy. Internal cleansing is required before rejuvenation and optimum health can be achieved.

Toxins accumulate in the organs and tissues of the body from eating animal-based foods, cooked and starchy foods and refined and processed foods. They also accumulate when inorganic multivitamin/mineral supplements are taken, for reasons that have already been discussed. The body also gets toxins from the environment, e.g., from exhaust fumes, municipal drinking water, etc.

When the body contains many poisons and is daily given more of them through the foods that are eaten, ill health reigns. When the body is cleansed of its toxins and is daily given living plant foods, health reigns.

Raw plant foods possess the highest level of nutrients found in any food, and bestow numerous health benefits, some of which are yet to be discussed in this book. An abundance of vitality is available to anyone who adopts the raw vegan diet. When toxins are removed from the body through the self-cleansing process that is enhanced by eating raw plant foods, you feel great.

What is known as "toxic overload" may occur when the detoxification/self-cleansing process is ramped into high gear by a sudden shift to an all whole plant food diet.

The sudden shift causes an abundance of toxins to be released into the bloodstream all at once, and, as confirmed by many raw food eaters and nutritional experts, this may cause flu or disease like symptoms to occur creating discomfort and malaise. People have gotten seriously ill from transitioning too quickly to the raw vegan diet. This is why a gradual transition to the raw vegan diet is recommended. The purpose of eating some cooked foods during the transition period is to slow down the detoxification process in order to avoid toxic overload.

Living plant foods are so powerful that they immediately start cleansing the body of its poisons. Their life force actions on the body drive out toxic wastes into the bloodstream for their elimination through the normal elimination organs of the body (including the skin). The powers of living plant foods are clearly evidenced by the signs the body gives when it detoxifies itself on these foods.

David Wolfe in his book, *The Sunfood Diet Success System*, states that detoxification stops when cooked food is eaten. The dangers associated with cooked foods, why they are detrimental to human health, are described in the chapter on "The Dangers of Cooked Foods."

Wastes released into the system from eating a whole plant food diet initially make you feel unhealthy, and during the self-cleansing process you may experience some signs of ill health. But that is natural and normal. It is caused by the toxins within the tissues and organs of the body being released into the bloodstream. Feelings of fatigue, dizziness, and the signs cited below may be experienced until the "house cleaning" is completed. But when the toxins are eliminated, the feeling of true health is experienced.

The possible ill effects of detoxification should not in any way dissuade the reader from proceeding with a whole plant food diet, since it is the way to true health. They are provided so that you will not be surprised by them when you undergo detoxification.

Normal signs of detoxification include: frequent urinations and/or bowel movements, diarrhea, headaches, runny nose, colds, expectoration, loss of energy, feelings of melancholy, needing more sleep, etc., all indications that the body is purging itself of toxins. Additional signs of detoxification are found in Robert Morse's book, *The Detox Miracle Sourcebook.*

We need to take detoxification into stride when we start eating raw plant foods exclusively. Continue through the healing process trusting that the body is gaining health by what it is doing. Know that drugs that block these symptoms also block the healing process.

The transient discomforts of detoxification cause some people to quit a whole plant food diet like the raw vegan diet before the benefits are obtained because they do not understand the detoxification process. But those who stick with the process experience the tremendous boost in vitality that follows self-cleansing, when the accumulated poisons are removed from the system.

"There is only one true healing modality – detoxification. It will bring the body's chemistry back into homeostasis (balance) and remove the toxic metals, elements and substances that don't belong there." - Robert Morse, N.D., The Detox Miracle Sourcebook.

Those who have never experienced detoxification cannot know what it is like. You can read about it in books, like this one, and in articles on the Web, but unless you have personally gone through it you will never know what it is like.

"A pure raw plant diet assists the body's cleansing efforts in the most natural way by eliminating any toxicity from entering the system and by simultaneously moving toxicity through the lymph and blood and out the body through the eliminating organs (the bowels, kidneys, liver, skin, sinuses and lungs). A purification of the diet enforces a self-healing and radical whole-body rejuvenation." - David Wolfe, The Sunfood Diet Success System.

In my opinion, the chief importance of detoxification is to relieve the body of the burden of all forms of constipation, to peel away the coating of paste-like plaque that has formed on the walls of the intestines after years of eating the wrong foods, foods that are detrimental to health (see the chapter on "The Dangers of Starchy Foods.")

One of the things I learned during my first year on the raw vegan diet that was not covered in the books listed in the Bibliography, was that improper, or bad, food combinations can cause not only stomachache, headache, heartburn, and flatulence, but also constipation.

Colonics and Enemas

"Death begins in the colon." - Elie Metchnikoff.

Nutritional experts contend that many of the problems we are now facing, including age-related health disorders, are due to the condition of our colons. But they go further and tell us that many, if not most, diseases of humankind originate in the colon. This incredible assertion is explained in the books by Arnold Ehret, Dr. Ann Wigmore and Dr. N. W. Walker that are listed in the Bibliography, and is supported by other nutritional experts.

Hippocrates said, "All disease begins in the gut."

"Your constitutional encumbrances throughout the entire system are the source of every disease; the greatest and most harmful source of lowered vitality, imperfect health, lack of strength and endurance and any and all imperfect conditions. All have their source in the colon, never perfectly emptied since your birth." - Arnold Ehret, The Mucusless Diet Healing System.

What if we acted on this information? If there is a direct link between the diseases of humankind and the condition of the colon, shouldn't we do whatever is possible to eliminate toxic waste buildup and the plate-out of the plaque in the colon? Of course we should, and each of us can.

Colonics and enemas help to remove the plaque-like deposits in our colons and release and move toxins out of our systems. In this way, they accelerate the self-cleansing and healing process of the body. Nutritional experts Arnold Ehret, Dr. Norman Walker and others consider colonics and enemas either highly advantageous or absolutely necessary for healing chronic diseases.

If you have never had a colonic or enema, you are not alone. Most people have never had them, and many have never even heard of them. However, as we journey to optimum health we become more and more our own doctors. The transition to the raw vegan diet is the time to learn what these procedures are and how to perform them.

Colonics (also known as colon irrigations or colon hydrotherapy), are procedures performed in the privacy of a personal suite at a local colonic establishment. They help clean out the toxins and wastes accumulated in the colon.

Colonic establishments are located in most cities. The average cost for a colonic irrigation (or hydrotherapy) ranges $60-$100 and you can purchase multiple sessions to save money. I have done the colon hydrotherapy several times. The machine is self-operated and easy to use. You can control it at your own pace for as long as you want. For me, that was about 30 minutes. I decided on the colonics after I read the books by Dr. N.W. Walker in the Bibliography, and particularly his book, *Become Younger*.

A less expensive way to help the detoxification process is to perform enemas at home. Enema kits are available at most retail stores (Wal-Mart, drug stores, etc.). Each kit has a number of small plastic bottles that contain a saline solution. The procedure is to lie down, turn on one side and insert the tip of the bottle and squeeze the bottle. I discovered that better results are obtained by replacing half of the saline solution with freshly-squeezed lemon juice, and using 2 bottles at a time instead of one.

Other types of enema kits are available, such as the travel-bag variety which consists of a long plastic tube and a plastic bag that can be hung from a door knob.

Doing enemas is a good, positive change to make in your life. It is a learning experience that many would much rather avoid, but again, you are becoming more and more your own doctor as you continue on the raw vegan journey.

If you have less than three bowel movements a day then you should be doing colonics and/or enemas on a more frequent basis than once a month. Otherwise, once a month is recommended.

Colonics and enemas are not coffee-table topics for discussion. They are real-world procedures that need to be understood if anyone is serious about achieving optimum health.

For a more thorough discussion of the need for colonics and enemas, see the books by Arnold Ehret and N.W. Walker in the Bibliography.

Remember, if optimum health and longevity required no knowledge or effort or discernment whatsoever on the part of the individual, then they would be easy to come by and everyone would have them. If optimum health could be sold as a magic pill or silver bullet, anyone could easily become healthy without the slightest effort, and this book would not be written. But all things are given to us at the expenditure of effort.

"The "basement" of the human "temple" is the reservoir from which every symptom of disease and weakness is supplied in all its manifestations." - Arnold Ehret, The Mucusless Diet Healing System.

If you actively incorporate the information contained in this chapter into your life, you will be doing your health a great service, and perhaps more than you may realize.

Fasting

I consider fasting to be instrumental to the attainment of optimum health, even if it means just skipping a meal occasionally or practicing a no-breakfast plan.

Fasting acts so powerfully on the body that many diseases can be completely cured through the practice of fasting alone. For this reason, I highly recommend that some form of fasting be practiced if the aim is to achieve and maintain optimum health.

If fasting can cure almost all human diseases, what does that tell us about how diseases and other health disorders originate? It clearly indicates that the principle cause of disease lies in the foods that are eaten, and it implicates many of our ailments with improper diet. This, of course, is what the nutritionists have been telling us for years.

Fasting is so significant to the attainment of genuine health that if the reader gets nothing out of this book but the importance of fasting, then the book will have served its purpose, because fasting signifies, and in the practice of fasting is found, almost all of the health principles that are elucidated in this book.

As explained in this chapter on transitioning to the raw vegan diet, many new things need to be learned on the journey to optimum health. Foremost among them are detoxification, colonics, enemas and fasting.

If you do not know how to do the things described in this chapter, but you seriously want to have the best of health, then you should learn how to do them. It is all part of the adventure.

"Our joy, our happiness is in growing." - Alfred Armand Montapert.

The Final Hurdle

This chapter covers how to clear the final hurdle to achieve the God-given diet, the raw vegan diet. Assuming the transition period is almost completed, you should be on the vegan diet. To attain the raw vegan diet, a last hurdle remains, the hurdle of overcoming the addiction to cooked foods.

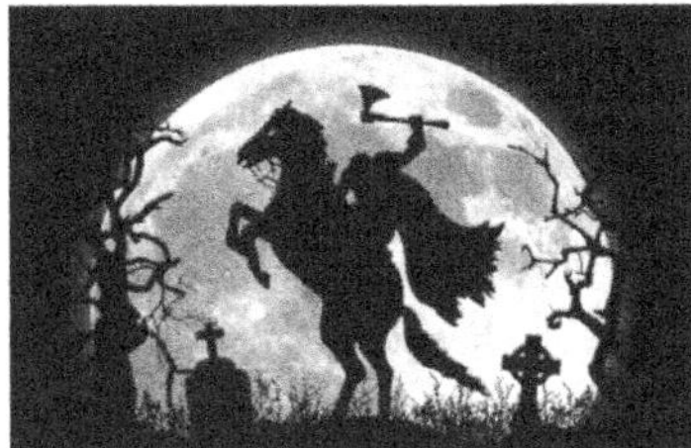

"Our deepest fear is not that we are inadequate. Our deepest fear is that we are powerful beyond measure. It is our light, not our darkness that most frightens us." - Marianne Williamson.

When I was on the vegan diet, I still ate cooked foods. The cooked foods I ate at the time of the final hurdle were canned beans and microwaved sweet potatoes, cabbage, broccoli and carrots. All other foods that I ate were raw fruits and vegetables, leafy greens, nuts and seeds, sea vegetables and Superfoods. The only thing that separated me from being a raw vegan was cooked food.

It was a struggle because my taste buds "knew better" and argued for keeping cooked foods in the diet. It was actually my cravings for cooked foods that stood in the way.

However, before I could get off cooked foods altogether, I had to be fully convinced that they were doing me harm. I had to understand the dangers that are inherent in eating cooked foods. It was part of my searching for the answers for why my health had reached a standstill and was no longer improving on the vegan diet.

I discovered that the dangers of cooked foods are best elucidated in the books by Norman W. Walker, Arnold Ehret and David Wolfe (see Bibliography). Some of the wisdom contained in these books has been captured in the previous chapters on "The Dangers of Cooked Foods" and "The Dangers of Starchy Foods." If these chapters have not convinced you of the dangers of eating these foods, then you should read the books that are referenced in those chapters. Remember that books are our most trusted source of information about foods and nutrition.

It was the knowledge of the dangers of cooked and starchy foods that enabled me to overcome the strong pulls and ties that these foods have on us. Otherwise, I would still be on the vegan diet, and still hindered by a partially healthy, partially unhealthy diet.

I believe that when you can conceptualize or visualize something, then it has a chance to manifest itself in your life. When I was convinced that cooked foods were harmful to my health, I quit them cold-turkey. It was the application of what I had learned over the power of the cravings I had for these foods. Then, all of a sudden, I was a raw vegan.

However, that did not end the battle that was waging between my taste buds and mind, as I was soon to find out.

My first day on the God-given diet was a red-letter day. I circled it on the calendar. I had at least made the decision to go completely raw.

The very first week of eating only raw plant foods passed quickly and uneventfully, to my great amazement. I was actually doing it; I was making it! I had some minor adjustments to make, to include more living foods in place of the dead foods I had been eating, but everything went well and I was learning more along the way. I circled each day on the calendar as time went by.

I remember it was very exciting. I guess I have always loved new challenges, and this was no exception. Soon, it was two whole weeks of eating only living plant foods. I couldn't believe that I was actually doing it! My self-confidence went up about fifty points.

In the third week of being totally raw, however, intense cravings for cooked foods surfaced and started to really bother me. My mouth would water just thinking about them. I began to second guess this whole raw food thing. After all, why should I give up foods that I really enjoy?? I would take a can of beans and just look at it. I would add more sweet potatoes to my shopping basket just to ensure I had enough at home, in case I started eating them again. It was a struggle that lasted all of the third week and persisted into the fourth week on the God-given diet.

To keep my mind from wondering, I put all cooked food items out of sight and kept the aforementioned books ready at hand, reading them over and over, and continuing to underline sentences that accentuated the dangers of cooked foods.

"When you're going through hell, keep going." - Winston Churchill.

The next thing I knew, a whole month had gone by on the raw vegan diet. The cravings for cooked foods passed along with it.

I discovered it actually *was* mind over matter, knowledge over desire. And that is how I overcame my cooked food addiction and cleared the hurdle.

I have not returned to cooked foods since and have no intention of doing so. When you are on the whole plant food God-given diet for any length of time, you no longer think about cooked foods. It turns out that nothing you lost was really worth keeping anyway.

How to Quit Cooked Foods

In addition to my own testimony given above, some objective advice and encouragement is warranted.

In order to quit cooked foods, to overcome their addictive power in your life, you must step out of your comfort zone one more time. It requires about the same amount of effort it took to quit meat and dairy products and all sugary foods.

First, there must be a resolve to quit cooked foods based on your self-education and knowledge about foods and nutrition. Then, you must summon the willpower to make it happen.

As mentioned in the chapter on "How Eating Habits are Formed," the so-called cravings of appetite are nothing more than ingrained habits. A habit once acquired and persistently practiced soon becomes a craving. There were no cravings until we acquired and persistently practiced a habit. Cravings stay with us even if they are doing us harm.

Anyone with a little persistence and willpower can change their eating habits, or for that matter any other habit in life. True change always begins in the mind. New eating habits are formed when we accustom the mind to new tastes and food selections based on reason and knowledge rather than emotional pulls and pressures.

"Uncooked foods will supply not only all the necessary vitamins and minerals, but also all the enzymes and easily digestible natural starches and proteins needed for healthy functioning of the body." - Paavo O. Airola, N.D., There is a Cure for Arthritis.

Food cravings, habits and addictions that are created or formed when the same foods are habitually eaten, are broken when the foods are continually not eaten. Begin the process by reducing the number of cooked foods in your diet and the frequency of eating them. When you reach a minimum of cooked foods in your diet, strengthen your resolve by reading as much as you can about the dangers of cooked foods and understanding why they are harmful to you.

Effort is required to accomplish anything worthwhile. The dictionary is the only place where success comes before work. Surely, nothing worthwhile in life is ever accomplished without effort, and the things that require the most effort are often the most rewarding and worthwhile of all.

The only way you will ever realize what it takes to quit cooked foods is by actually quitting them. No one can do it for you, it has to be done by you.

As mentioned previously, there is no magic pill or silver bullet for getting well. If you want anything to happen in life, you have to make it happen. That includes quitting cooked foods.

If the raw vegan diet were easy to attain and had zero hurdles to overcome, then more people would be experiencing its remarkable health benefits, and a lot less of the population would be rushing blindly towards premature graves.

The easy way is always the most traveled, and the difficult way is always the least travelled.

"Enter by the narrow gate; for wide is the gate and broad is the way that leads to destruction, and there are many who go in by it. Because narrow is the gate and difficult is the way which leads to life, and there are few who find it." - Jesus in the Bible, Matt. 7:13-14.

Afterwards

You have now successfully transitioned to the raw vegan diet. Congratulations! You have achieved what few people will ever accomplish. Your determination, discipline and willpower are to be commended. The efforts that you have made will now pay off.

Once the basics of the whole plant food diet are understood (and they are understood when they are put into practice), you have at your disposal the most potent healing and transformational tool ever available. And that is when the adventure really begins.

On a whole plant food diet, self-cleansing is in full gear. The self-cleansing process begins internally and is then reflected externally. This goes against conventional wisdom which says that to be clean all you must do is thoroughly wash with soap and water, but that only contributes to external cleansing. Internal cleansing is necessary to remove the toxins and pasty crud that have accumulated in the organs and tissues of the body from years of eating cooked and starchy foods and other foods and food products that are harmful to health. Normal signs of detoxification, previously discussed, are likely to be experienced, especially as more raw fruits and vegetables are eaten.

The skin, and particularly the skin of the face, reflects our internal health condition. A bad skin complexion (e.g., pimples or blotches on the face) indicates internal poisoning. A clear complexion reveals internal health. It doesn't take long on the raw vegan diet for the skin of the face to clear up, and then become smoother.

It has been reported by some raw food eaters that the face has actually takes on a perceptible glow or shine. This was revealed to me, for example, during a discussion I had with a raw food eater years ago who said he knew a man whose face actually glowed with health. I can't claim glowing skin, but I perceive that it is a possibility. After all, living plant foods provide us with their electric and magnetic properties intact, unaltered by heat. Also, isn't light a manifestation of electromagnetic energy?

Many Medieval and earlier Christian paintings, stained-glass windows and mosaics depict Jesus and the saints with halos over their heads. Could these depictions be based on fact? Arnold Ehret in his book, *The Cause and Cure of Human Illness*, states that many saints of old were self-radiant due to their ascetic diet of raw plant foods and their practice of fasting.

The thought of discovering the "Fountain of Youth" has intrigued many people for centuries, and there have been explorers, such as Ponce de Leon, who have tried to find it. I believe the fountain of youth exists, but not hidden in some distant, exotic land. I believe it is within every person, just waiting to be released through a diet of living plant foods.

Some people spend large amounts of money on beauty products and preparations. If the money were spent instead on self-education about foods and nutrition, and on raw, organic fruits, vegetables, leafy greens and other living plant foods, it would allow health and youthful appearance to be attained without the aid of these products.

Want to look young? Eat raw plant foods. Want to look old? Eat cooked foods.

Health improvements reported by raw food eaters the world over have included not only the complete healing of diseases, but changes indicative of rejuvenation, such as wrinkles disappearing, improved vision, hair growing back and hair color returning to that of former years, among other things. These signs, while seemingly miraculous, are logical consequences of eating living plant foods once you understand the healing powers of these foods. Such improvements are due to the life force in raw plant foods, life force made available to anyone on the raw began diet.

On the raw vegan diet, the body is cleansed not only of poisonous substances that have accumulated over the years and have been deposited deeply in body tissues, but also those that get into the body from the environment, or from foods and drinks, such as chlorine and heavy metals from municipal drinking water, pesticides in non-organic produce, and tobacco and alcohol use.

"Any substance, when taken into the body, is either a food or a poison." - Dr. Herbert M. Shelton, Superior Nutrition.

Modern nutritional experts believe that fruits and leafy green vegetables are the greatest cleansers of the body. Both food groups cause toxins to be released from the tissues. The more fruits and leafy greens we eat on a regular basis, the more our internals are scrubbed clean and the more our outward improvements are manifested. Since the self-cleansing process will be on-going from now on, so will visible health improvements.

The effectiveness of the self-cleansing process is also evident by the composition, odor and frequency of stools. Bowel movements become smoother, less smelly and more frequent, which are all signs of internal cleansing becoming a more normal process, and indicating a less clogged up condition due to better digestion and the ongoing removal of poisons from the body. On the raw vegan diet, you may find that the number of bowel movements per day is at least as many as the number of meals eaten per day. Constipation is unknown on the raw vegan diet.

The secret of vitality is found in raw plant foods. An abundance of vitality is available to anyone who adopts the raw vegan diet.

The nutritional experts agree that the raw vegan diet, together with fasting, dissolves accumulated toxins better than any other health regimen. When toxins are removed from the body, you feel great.

If you wake up in the mornings feeling groggy, sluggish and in a sour mood, it is probably because of accumulated poisons and waste material that still reside in you, not only in your colon but in the very tissues of your body. These poisons can be adequately purged by eating living plant foods, watching our intake of harmful foods and drinks, performing enemas or colonics and fasting.

The Benefits

Based on my experience and the experiences of others, I believe that the raw vegan diet provides more benefits than have been accounted for or recognized, and that the benefits are boundless, as Nature is boundless.

When I was a vegetarian, and also when I was a vegan, I had health issues that simply could not be shaken. They remained with me until I became a raw vegan. I was plagued with chronic fatigue. I felt worn-out all the time despite getting sufficient sleep. I took organic iron supplements, sublingual vitamin B12 spray, flaxseeds, chia seeds and kelp to counter this condition, but they did not solve the problem.

After being on the raw vegan diet for only a short time, my fatigue vanished into thin air. I now have a surplus of energy. I never have to lie down during the day or take a nap anymore.

"Most persons are tired because their body lacks enzymes. The food they eat cannot be utilized constructively but is turned instead into toxins, poisons which lead to sickness. Enzymes, apparently, are the key to longevity; they seem to neutralize the basic causes of aging and enable the body to retain its youthful qualities." - Dr. Ann Wigmore, Be Your Own Doctor.

I attribute the fatigue that I had prior to the raw vegan diet to the lack of enzymes in the cooked foods I was eating. After several years on the diet, however, I decided it might be wise to take, as a precaution, sublingual vitamin B12 because of the fact that a lack of vitamin B12 is considered a possibility when eating raw plant foods exclusively. But I now never take it.

I had scaly skin on the karate edges of my hands every winter, from November through March. On the raw vegan diet, this condition disappeared.

I'm more physically fit and active now than I've been in years. I lost 14 pounds going from the vegan diet to the raw vegan diet. That's 14 pounds I no longer have to carry around. Also, my vision has improved. I can read books outdoors without corrective lenses. The last time I could do that was in my 40s.

I've had a number of physical ailments including hemorrhoids, sciatica, spinal stenosis and arthritis. But since being on the diet, I have had no further health issues and, of course, no diseases. I cured my hemorrhoids by a simple plant food remedy that is not well known. It is described in the book on hemorrhoids in the Bibliography. I cured my sciatica and spinal stenosis through correction of muscle imbalances as explained in the book on sciatica and spinal stenosis in the Bibliography. I tried so many things to cure my arthritis that I know that the diet, distilled water and intermittent fasting are what have resulted in no more pains.

However, the health improvements I received on the diet pale into insignificance compared to the health improvements experienced by many other raw plant food eaters, including nutritional experts Arnold Ehret, O.L.M. Abramowski, Ann Wigmore, Norman W. Walker, Bernard Jensen, Herbert M. Shelton, Theresa Mitchell, David Wolfe, Professor Spira, Harvey Diamond, Kristina Carrillo-Bucaram, Victoria Boutenko, Tonya Zavasta, and Joe Alexander. Some of these individuals were but a step away from death before they cured themselves of serious chronic diseases through the raw vegan diet. Some also healed themselves of other conditions through the diet, such as bursitis (Tonya Zavasta), and colitis and arthritis (Ann Wigmore). Their testimonies are included in their books listed in the Bibliography. They validate the power of living plant foods to completely heal illnesses and diseases.

I highly recommend the books in the Bibliography just for the testimonies. They will convince you of the importance of eating living plant foods exclusively, and encourage you in the diet.

It may interest you to know that Norman W. Walker lived to be 99 (according to the Web), but some sources, including David Wolf, say 109. Herbert M. Shelton lived to be 100. Dr. Bernard Jensen lived to be 93. Dr. Edward Howell lived to 90. Dr. D. C. Jarvis lived to 85. Arnold Ehret died accidentally at 56 when he slipped on a wet, oil-soaked street in California and fell back and hit his head on the payment. Dr. Ann Wigmore died at 85 from smoke inhalation when a fire broke out at her Institute while she was sleeping. Most of the other nutritional experts are still living.

The body is the greatest healing machine. It only requires the right foods to accomplish what it alone knows how to do. When living plant foods are eaten in place of dead, cooked foods, the body receives the amazing ionic and magnetic properties of living foods as well as their potent, unaltered natural minerals, vitamins and enzymes.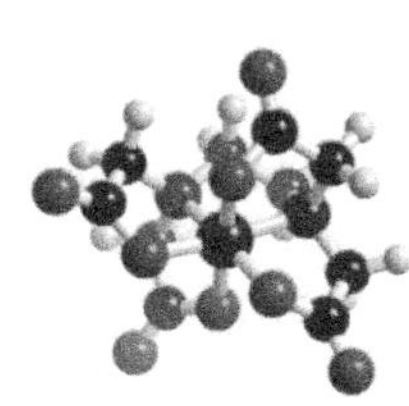

The on-going self-cleansing of the body that is achieved by eating living plant foods exclusively is complemented by another process, one that is also on-going. That process is the cellular reconstruction of the body.

The body is constantly replacing its cells. Old cells are being replaced by new cells. The difference between the raw vegan diet and other diets is that on the raw vegan diet the body is provided with the best raw materials for this reconstruction process.

When we eat cooked foods including refined and processed man-made foods, which are dead foods, the new cells are constructed of inferior quality building materials.

"Dead atoms and dead molecules cannot rejuvenate or regenerate the cells of the body. Such food results in cell starvation and this in turn causes sickness and disease." - Norman W. Walker, Water Can Undermine Your Health.

The time required for cellular reconstruction varies depending on the organs and tissues of the body. The following information is taken from the Web.

AVERAGE BODY CELL REPLACEMENT TIME

- White blood cells   2-5 days

- Stomach cells   2-9 days

- Lung alveoli   8 days

- Trachea cells   1-2 months

- Red blood cells   5 months

- Skeleton cells   10% p.a.

This indicates that after only a short time, the body has replaced many of its cells, and if we are on the raw vegan diet the new cells have been made from the best raw materials of life, those found in living plant foods. The longer we eat raw foods exclusively, the more we are being reconstructed from the materials provided by living plant foods.

It requires years for the body to replace all of its cells (which number some ten trillion), but, in time, they all get replaced – at least the vast majority of them do as far as we know. It is uncertain whether all the neurons of the brain get replaced.

Some scientists believe that at any one time in a person's life, the cells and tissues of the body are no more than 7 years old. If true, it sets a short-term goal for all of us on the raw vegan diet, which is to remain on the diet for at least 7 years to be totally reconstructed from the best raw materials of Nature.

The new you is in the making, and you are able to sense it, and that alone makes each day a new experience. You are being transformed inside out, and if you pause for a moment during your busy day to think about it, it just may put a smile on your face.

As discussed previously, the raw vegan diet provides all the vitamins, proteins, and other nutrients required to attain and sustain a healthy life. However, some raw foodists have reported a deficiency of vitamin B-12. There are few plant foods that contain vitamin B-12. To be on the safe side, you can take a vitamin B-12 supplement in the form of an organic sublingual spray, which is available at whole food stores. As with all of the B vitamins, vitamin B-12 is water soluble and flushes out of the system if more is taken than the body can use. You can also take an organic iron supplement to help avoid fatigue.

If you take supplements, you should ensure that they are in organic, not inorganic, form. As explained previously, the cells of the body utilize minerals that are in organic form, which is one of the reasons that plant foods are so important to us. Plants convert the inorganic minerals found in the soil and water into organic form that is readily assimilated by the body.

A noticeable improvement occurred after time on the diet. My senses of smell and taste became keener, which helped me to refine and improve my diet, such as by eating more nutritious raw plant foods and avoiding ones not so nutritious.

The only "shock" I experienced on the raw vegan diet occurred several months into the diet. I noticed many large wrinkles on my skin, especially on the face and the back of the neck. My immediate reaction was, what is going on? So once again, I went to books for the answers. I discovered that this occurrence is normal on the raw vegan diet, and that it soon passes. It is reflective of the detoxification process and indicates the success of it. Teresa Mitchell explains this in her book, *My Road to Health*. She states that it is a normal sign of the healing process that is going on. The wrinkles go away and skin elasticity returns when the blood and tissues are rebuilt using the optimum building blocks of living natural foods. And that is exactly what happened to me.

As for habits such as alcohol and tobacco, the diet will eventually cause the body to reject what is bad for it. If you have difficulty quitting such habits, then let the diet handle it for you.

SAY GOODBYE TO THESE THINGS

- Microwave Oven

- Stove

- Baking Accessories

- Pots and Pans

- Cooking Utensils

- Can Openers

- Popcorn Maker

- Toaster

- Rice Cooker

The same week I quit cooked foods and became a raw vegan, I gave away my microwave oven. By giving it away, I burned a bridge to my past that I never want to cross again. When I was convinced of the harmful effects that cooked foods have on the body, I wanted to be not only free of cooked foods, but of all the devices or gadgets I possessed which were used in connection with cooked foods.

Getting rid of the microwave oven and the other cooking tools and utensils was my declaration of independence on the raw vegan diet. It cemented my resolve to stick with the diet.

The stove, because of its bulk and weight, was more difficult to give away, so I kept it. It now has a large cutting board spanning the upper burners. I sometimes use the oven in winter to help heat up the kitchen. Otherwise, it goes unused.

In addition, canned, bottled or jarred food products in the kitchen cabinets can now be given away or donated to the local food banks, many of which are supported by local churches that have drop off centers you can use.

The new-found space in the kitchen can then be put to better use for storage of raw food items, such as containers of nuts and seeds, sun-dried fruits and Superfoods.

Specific Benefits of the Raw Vegan Diet

Some of the benefits of the raw vegan diet have already been described. Below is a more complete list. These benefits have been experienced by raw food eaters in every generation the world over, including myself and the authors of the books that are listed in the Bibliography. The benefits are all extraordinary in their own way. Some are experienced after only a short time on the diet.

- Heals diseases

- Prevents diseases from taking root in the body

- Rejuvenates and beautifies

- Increases energy

- Promotes health and longevity

- Reduces weight

- Improves mental clarity

- Adds excitement to life

- Improves decision making

- Improves sleeps

- Makes you feel good about being alive

Let's examine two that have not yet been discussed.

Let's take the last benefit first. How many people do you know, or see every day, who have a frown on their face? How many times can that be said of you? Our general health affects the way that we feel, which often results in a display of outward signs. When we are healthy, we feel good about being alive and tend to show it. When we're unhealthy, we tend to show that too.

Raw plant foods enhance the spirit in definite ways, charging or supercharging it. After about a year on the diet, you will find yourself paying more attention to the spiritual aspects of life than before, perhaps praying more often and earnestly than you did before, because you are thankful for being given the life that you have.

The healing of diseases is the most significant benefit that can be expected on the raw vegan diet. As explained previously, healing is achieved by eating living raw plant foods exclusively, adopting proper eating habits, and performing fasting. It is the natural consequence of the on-going cellular reconstruction process utilizing the best building materials found in Nature, and the bodily detoxification process that follows.

"All illnesses, including the inherited diseases, stem from biologically wrong, unnatural food, and from every gram of excess food intake. The exceptions are rare, e.g., lack of hygiene." - Arnold Ehret, The Mucusless Diet Healing System.

How long does it take for healing to occur on the raw vegan diet? According to the nutritional experts, it depends on how long one has been eating harmful foods. Many people have neglected their health for years before becoming a raw vegan.

The healing process can be speeded up depending on what is done to assist it. For example, if you periodically fast and perform colonics and/or enemas, then quicker results can be expected. If you do not do these things, then delayed results can be expected. But the important thing is, the healing process begins in earnest when you are committed to the raw vegan diet.

David Wolfe in his book, *The Sunfood Diet Success System*, states that it typically takes one month on the diet to reverse one year on a cooked/toxic food diet, to dissolve and eliminate the improper materials that have accumulated in the body. But this schedule, apparently, does not consider the accelerators of periodic fasting and colonics and/or enemas.

The excitement builds as progress becomes more noticeable on the diet. For example, in a very short time on the raw vegan diet you will begin to lose weight. Also, your complexion will clear up. Other encouraging rejuvenation signs will appear as well.

Expect to have a surplus of energy that enables you to do more things. Expect to be able to work and play without tiring.

You will begin to function at an enhanced awareness level. Your senses of sight, sound, smell and taste will become more acute, or heightened.

You will have a clarity of mind that will enable you to make right decisions.

You will sense that more health improvements are on the way. You realize that the days ahead are going to be better than the days behind. Isn't that how you want to start every day of your life?

As the health improvements become more apparent, you will be able to gauge your progress. But, however long it takes, do not give up.

The more you can hone, or attune, the diet to the preferences of the body, the healthier you will become, and the sharper your mind will become. In particular, you learn to avoid foods that are difficult to digest.

"As your body becomes smarter and more accustomed to the changes you are introducing, it will direct you toward consuming less food, and that food will be of the very best quality. No matter how incredible it might sound to a beginner, the day will come when you will no longer care for recipes. At first you cannot stand the lightness that consumption of raw foods produces, but after several years on this lifestyle it is fullness that becomes insufferable." - Tonya Zavasta, <u>Beautiful on Raw Uncooked Creations</u>.

I am more convinced now than ever before that the most beneficial plant foods, those that contribute most to the healing process and to optimum health, are the foods that are the most "alive," that is, foods that have been the most recently harvested.

Many, if not all, of the raw plant foods that are sold in local food stores have been harvested more than a week ago (unless grown locally). They have been shipped-in from faraway places in an un-ripened condition, which typically means that they have been in cold storage for weeks. They have been sprayed with wax to retard spoilage. They have been labeled. Most appear to be flawless copies of one other, uniform in size, shape and color.

Locally grown and/or Community Supported Agriculture (CSA) farm produce is organically grown produce. The farms are typically family owned and operated, or non-profit organizations. The produce is typically no more than a few days old from being harvested at peak ripeness. It hasn't been labelled or sprayed with wax. CSA fruits and vegetables are not necessarily uniform in appearance, but they typically have flaws. Their life-giving properties have been least altered or affected by the growers and the suppliers.

I benefit from a CSA and recommend everyone do the same. If you happen to live in a country other than the US, there should be a local food producer and supplier in your area where fresh produce is available.

In my opinion, the further away we get from the heavy use of herbicides and pesticides in the many large-scale factory farms, the prematurely harvested foods that are shipped-in from long distances, such as from China, South America and Africa, and the various cosmetic measures that have been applied to them to make them more appealing to the sight, the better off we will be as consumers of fruits, vegetables and other raw foods, and the quicker we will experience the benefits of the raw vegan diet.

"I believe that family farms ought to be considered our greatest natural resource, and that the fundamental healthfulness of our food and the long-term health of our economy are closely tied to their well-being." - Howard F. Lyman, Mad Cowboy.

The nutritional advantages of eating locally grown produce over other produce have been covered in the chapter on "What Foods Should We Eat and Why?"

Most of us lack the yard space for planting a garden, and only few of us will ever be able to afford a farm. The closest most of us will ever get to locally grown produce is by joining a CSA.

We have spent too much time and effort learning about the foods of the animal kingdom and how to prepare them. It is time we learned about the foods of the plant kingdom and the many tasty and nutritious meals that can be made from them. Each kind of living plant food has its own unique blend of nutrients and life-giving properties. We can benefit from eating many types of raw plant foods. I believe that vast variety of plant foods in the world have been given to us for a purpose, and that we can discover that purpose by becoming familiar with these foods.

An aspect of a whole plant food diet that strikes me as being perhaps the most interesting is that it doesn't leave you guessing about whether your health is going to improve. Your health does not stall or level-off and then decline on the diet, as it does on other diets. It continues to improve. Each day on the diet is an ongoing progression, a new adventure, sometimes trying until the key points discussed in this book are mastered, but never a losing proposition. Each day that you are on the diet you are a winner.

A new story is being written. It is a story that continues to be written as long as you remain on the living food, raw vegan diet. It is a story about you – the new you. Maybe it is the best story ever.

"Let food be thy medicine and medicine be thy food." - Hippocrates.

"Let food be thy medicine and medicine be thy food." - Hippocrates.

Next Steps

I encourage you to read the books listed in the Bibliography. They have much to offer the novice as well as the long-time student of foods and nutrition. We all like to eat, but it is only when we learn to eat foods that promote health, not destroy it, that our health flourishes. The books provide valuable information and inspiration that will help all seekers of health. They have been a constant source of encouragement to me on my health journey. Take the time to delve into them and you will be glad that you did.

The feelings of exuberance and goodness that are hallmarks of a whole plant food diet, like the raw vegan diet, are the result of eating the right foods and combining foods properly. The opposite feelings are experienced on ordinary diets resulting from poor nutrition, poor digestion, toxic waste accumulation and constipation. The life force properties that are in raw plant foods make all the difference.

In Closing

As more and more fad diets, miracle treatments and supplements become available and attract the attention of millions, so are more and more people throughout the world discovering the health advantages of eating at variance with the customs of the times, and the simple truth that eating natural plant foods leads to good health. They are taking back responsibility for their health and abandoning culturally accepted foods. Truly, these are the lucky ones.

At this very moment, the cells of your body are changing, and the building materials used for that process are the best there are if you are on the raw vegan diet. The advantages of eating raw plant foods are immeasurable, both to us and our progeny.

However, the times require vigilance if we wish to maintain the great strides that have been made in the availability of raw fruits and vegetables, and organic plant foods. We are being thrust into a future that may not be health-wise beneficial for us. We need to keep an eye out for what's ahead, what's around the corner. If raw plant foods (for human consumption) begin to be big business, the meat-, grain- and dairy-based interests may feel threatened and apply pressure on the producers and suppliers of these foods. Hopefully, that is a long way off. it seems at least that raw plant foods may never cause a mass exodus away from the typical American diet.

One of the greatest physicists, Max Planck, said that over the temple of science should be written the words, "Ye must have faith." The great apostle Paul wrote to his new church in Thessalonica, "Prove all things; hold fast that which is good." A scientist says, "Have faith." A saint says "Prove all things." Together, they spell HOPE.

Bibliography

The following books are the major resources used to write this book.

1. T. Colin Campbell, <u>The China Study</u>, 2006.

2. Dr. Michael Greger, <u>How Not To Die</u>, 2015.

3. John Smith, Fruits and Farinacea- <u>The Proper Food of Man</u>, 2015.

4. Russell T. Trall, <u>Scientific Basis of Vegetarianism</u>, 1970.

5. Dr. Caldwell Esselstyn, Jr., <u>Prevent and Reverse Heart Disease</u>, 2007.

6. Jethro Kloss, <u>Back to Eden</u>, 2014.

7. Dr. Ann Wigmore, <u>Be Your Own Doctor</u>, 1982.

8. Dr. Ann Wigmore, <u>Why You Do Not Have to Grow Old</u>, 1985.

9. Dr. Ann Wigmore, <u>The Sprouting Book</u>, 1986.

10. O. L. M. Abramowski, <u>Fruitarian Diet and Physical Rejuvenation</u>, 1916.

11. Arnold Ehret, <u>The Mucusless Diet Healing System</u>, 2015.

12. Arnold Ehret, <u>Rational Fasting and Roads to Health and Happiness</u>, 2002.

13. Arnold Ehret, <u>The Cause and Cure of Human Illness</u>, 2001.

14. Teresa Mitchell, <u>My Road to Health</u>, 1987.

15. Norman W. Walker, <u>Colon Health</u>, 2005.

16. Norman W. Walker, <u>Become Younger</u>, 1978.

17. Norman W. Walker, <u>Fresh Vegetable and Fruit Juices</u>, 1978.

18. Norman W. Walker, <u>Diet and Salad Suggestions</u>, 1985.

19. Norman W. Walker, <u>Water Can Undermine Your Health</u>, 1995.

20. Norman W. Walker, <u>The Natural Way to Vibrant Health</u>, 1972.

21. Victoria Boutenko, <u>Green for Life</u>, 2005.

22. Victoria Boutenko, <u>12 Steps to Raw Foods</u>, 2005.

23. David Wolfe, <u>The Sunfood Diet Success System</u>, 2008.

24. David Wolfe, <u>Longevity Now: A Comprehensive Approach</u>, 2013.

25. David Wolfe, <u>Superfoods, the Food and Medicine of the Future</u>, 2009.

26. Harvey Diamond, <u>Fit for Life Not Fat for Life</u>, 2003.

27. Harvey Diamond, <u>Living Without Pain</u>, 2007.

28. Dr. D. C. Jarvis, <u>Folk Medicine</u>, 1958.

29. D. C. Jarvis, <u>Arthritis & Folk Medicine</u>, 1960.

30. Robert O. Young and Shelly R. Young, <u>The pH Miracle</u>, 2010.

31. Paul C. and Patricia Bragg, <u>Apple Cider Vinegar, Miracle Health System</u>, 2008.

32. Paul C. and Patricia Bragg, <u>The Miracle of Fasting</u>, 2005

33. Dr. Edward Howell, <u>Enzyme Nutrition</u>, 1985.

34. Paul C. and Patricia Bragg, <u>Water, The Shocking Truth That Can Save Your Life</u>, 2004.

35. Edmond Bordeaux Szekely (Translator), <u>The Essene Gospel of Peace, Book One</u>, 1981.

36. Professor Spira, <u>Spira Speaks, Dialogs and Essays on The Mucusless Diet Healing System,</u> 2014.

37. Dr. Bernard Jensen, <u>Guide to Diet and Detoxification</u>, 2000.

38. Dr. Bernard Jensen, <u>The Healing Power of Chlorophyll</u>, 1973.

39. Fred S. Hirsch, Internal Cleanliness, 1987.

40. Tonya Zavasta, Beautiful on Raw Uncooked Creations, 2005.

41. Kristina Carrillo-Bucaram, The Fully Raw Diet, 2016.

42. Karyn Calabrese, Soak Your Nuts, 2011.

43. Herbert M. Shelton, Superior Nutrition, 1994.

44. Herbert M. Shelton, Fasting Can Save Your Life, 1978.

45. Herbert M. Shelton, Food Combining Made Easy, 1982.

46. Dr. Russel Blaylock, Excitotoxins, The Taste that Kills, 1997.

47. Joe Alexander, Blatant Raw Foodist Propaganda, 2005.

48. Horst Kornberger, Global Hive: Bee Crisis and Compassionate Ecology, 2012.

49. Steve Meyerowitz, Sprouts, The Miracle Food, 1997.

50. Dr. Henry Lindlahr, Philosophy of Natural Therapeutics, 1975.

51. Dan Georgakas, The Methuselah Factors, 1980.

52. Alexander Leaf, M.D., Youth in Old Age, 1975.

53. Andrew Weil, M.D,, Healthy Aging, 2005.

54. Luigi Cornaro, Sure Methods of Attaining a long and Healthful Life, 1660.

55. Luigi Cornaro, The Surest Method of Correcting An Infirm Constitution, 1660.

56. Luigi Cornaro, How to Live 100 Years, or Discourses on the Sober Life, 1660.

57. Dr. Johnny Lovewisdom, Dietetics Vitarianism, 2001.

58. Gabriel Cousens, M.D., Conscious Eating, 2000.

59. Jeffery M. Smith, <u>Genetic Roulette</u>, 2007.

60. F. Batmanghelidj, M.D, <u>Your Body's Many Cries for Water</u>, 2008.

61. Dr. Allen E. Banik, <u>The Choice is Clear</u>, 1989.

62. Robert Morse, N.D., <u>The Detox Miracle Sourcebook</u>, 2004.

63. Arnold Paul De Vries, <u>Therapeutic Fasting</u>, 1958

64. Dr. Kristine Nolfi, M.D., <u>The Miracle of Living Foods</u>, 1981.

65. T. Colin Campbell and Howard Jacobson, <u>Whole: Rethinking the Science of Nutrition</u>, 2014.

66. Wallace D. Wattles, <u>Health Through New Thought and Fasting</u>, 2007.

67. Francoise Wilhelmi de Toledo, MD, and Hubert Hohler, <u>Therapeutic Fasting: The Buchinger Amplius Method</u>, 2018.

68. Edward Hooker Dewey, M.D., <u>The No-Breakfast Plan and the Fasting Cure</u>. 1900.

69. Edward Hooker Dewey, M.D., <u>The True Science of Living</u>. 1894.

70. Upton Sinclair, <u>The Fasting Cure</u>, 1911.

71. Hereward Carrington, <u>Vitality, Fasting and Nutrition</u>, 1908.

72. Paavo O. Airola, N.D., <u>There is a Cure for Arthritis,</u> 1968.

73. Alfred Armand Montapert, <u>The Supreme Philosophy of Man: The Laws of Life</u>, 1977.

74. Stephen R. Covey, <u>The 7 Habits of Highly Effective People</u>, 2004.

75. Herbert M. Shelton, <u>Health for the Millions</u>, 1968.

76. Stan Shepherd, <u>How to Really Get Rid of Hemorrhoids, Naturally: A Permanent Cure</u>, 2018.

77. Stan Shepherd, <u>Stop Sciatica and Spinal Stenosis</u>, 2019.

About the Author

Stan Shepherd, 70, has researched and studied the human health field for over 30 years. An engineer by training, he has witnessed the rapid decline of health in this country over the years due to commonly eaten foods. The vital importance of telling others about the many health hazards associated with commonly eaten foods has been the incentive for writing this book.

Biographical:

I grew up in Michigan during the 50's and 60's. I witnessed the fervid race to the moon as well as the initial establishment of the fast food chains. When I was in grade school, my sandwiches were made of boloney or olive loaf slices between two mustard-spread slices of white Wonder Bread. My lunch box included a thermos for milk, but I usually bought a small carton of chocolate milk at the vending machines and a mini-bag of chips or Fritos. I ate what my parents ate and what was advertised on TV. Breakfast was usually Corn Pops, Sugar Pops, Chex, Cheerios, Wheaties, etc., with milk and table sugar. Dinner was often Swanson's TV Dinners. I can't remember seeing a salad during my growing up years except maybe at a restaurant. Dessert was typically ice cream, pie, cake or pudding. On weekends, breakfast could be bacon and eggs, or sausage and eggs, with white toast and jam or jelly, or pancakes or waffles with butter or margarine and syrup. For road trips, lunch was McDonald's or Burger King hamburgers or cheeseburgers, with fries and a coke or shake. The local Dairy Queen had creamy chocolate cones that weighed about a pound.

This gives the reader some idea of the American foodscape at the time I was growing up. Has anything really changed since then?

Had I been raised in a family that practiced a different kind of diet, such as a whole plant food diet, I'm sure I would have learned to eat healthier foods at an early age. That not being the case, I had to learn about foods and nutrition on my own.

Index

A

B

C

H

Hemp seed, 35, 40, 62-63.

Heart disease, 12-13, 39, 49.

Honey, 36-37, 41.

I

Inorganic minerals, 15-16, 70-74, 77-78, 89, 108.

Iodine, 31-32.

iron supplements, 104, 108.

K

Kidney disease (trouble), 36, 53, 75.

L

Legumes, 11, 24-25, 28, 37.

Longevity, 12, 19, 66-69, 83, 93, 104, 110.

M

Maca, 38-39, 62-64.

MSG, Monosodium Glutamate, 17.

N

Neurological disease, 18.

Nutrient deficiency, 15, 17, 54-55.

Nuts, 11, 14, 25, 28-30, 35, 41, 61, 110.

O

Obesity, 49.

Oils, fractionated, 39.

ORAC rating, 38.

T

U

V

Made in United States
North Haven, CT
24 April 2024

51710592R00072